# THE ANXIETY PROJECT

*Daan Heerma van Voss*

# THE ANXIETY PROJECT

A Journey to the Centre of Our Deepest Fears

*Translated from the Dutch by*
*David Doherty*

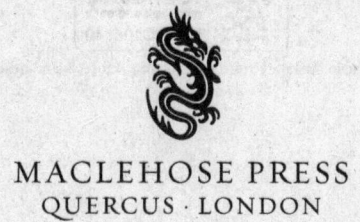

MACLEHOSE PRESS
QUERCUS · LONDON

First published in the Dutch language as *De bange mens*
by Uitgeverij Atlas Contact, Amsterdam in 2021
First published in Great Britain in 2023 by MacLehose Press
This paperback edition published in 2024 by

MacLehose Press
an imprint of Quercus Editions Ltd
Carmelite House
50 Victoria Embankment
London EC4Y 0DZ

An Hachette UK Company

The publisher gratefully acknowledges the support of the Dutch Foundation for Literature

**N**ederlands
**letterenfonds**
dutch foundation
for literature

A CIP catalogue record for this book is available
from the British Library.

ISBN (MMP) 978 1 52942 183 5
ISBN (Ebook) 978 1 52942 186 6

10 9 8 7 6 5 4 3 2

Designed and typeset in Scala by CC Book Production
Printed and bound in Great Britain by Clays Ltd, Elcograf S.p.A.

MIX
Paper | Supporting
responsible forestry
FSC® C104740

Papers used by MacLehose Press are from well-managed forests and other responsible sources.

# THE ANXIETY PROJECT

# Contents

For M.

# I

# *Red Lilies*

I hand her the flowers and she starts to cry. Slow tears. We are standing in the kitchen, this room we have built for ourselves – shelf by shelf, drawer by drawer – in the five years and more that we have been together. Sobbing quietly, she takes a knife and trims the stems; brisk taps on the chopping block. Afraid of what's coming, I stare at the fridge, at snapshots of recently married friends, cards announcing the arrival of children who now know our names. Lives we are part of. It made us smile to think we might be stuck on other people's fridges one day.

D. tells me how desperate she's been feeling these past weeks. She selects words that carry no blame, but there can be no mistake: I am the cause. I listen shamefaced to her vignettes of my behaviour; only the one you love can deliver an anamnesis as clear and as painful. I barely sleep, crave reassurance, dread leaving the house for every appointment. When I do step outside, it's hood up and eyes down. At night my teeth chatter; in the morning I wake up jittery and damp with sweat. She gets out of bed and I plead with her to stay a while, a little longer, just a few minutes more. Evening brings a semblance of relief at having made it through another day – an accomplishment I appear to think deserves some kind of medal.

But I am *functioning*, right?

She doesn't think so.

"I make it to my appointments, don't I?"

"Once you've had your daily panic attack on the stairs."

"You can hear that?"

She raises an eyebrow. I know she can hear it when my breath comes quick and shallow; she knows I know. Maybe I hope she'll pop her head round the door. Maybe I can't help myself. Am I just seeking attention?

"It's got to the stage when you're scared to set foot in your own study."

She's right. I've spent too long living for my work. The euphoria of meeting another deadline, the dopamine rush, lured me into accepting each new assignment. And when I recognised the pattern, my response was to rise above it and take on even more work. Then one day, a few months ago, I stopped dead in my tracks. There were no new plans, no ideas, but there was no rest either, not even boredom. No concentration and no relaxation. Only a haunted inertia, a spinning of the wheels that brought nothing but exhaustion. Friends with steady lives suggested hobbies like chopping wood or DIY and looked at me expectantly. I was reluctant to keep bringing up my feelings and, as every other topic of conversation began to feel trite or divorced from reality, I spoke less in company. D. said she thought it was a shame people didn't get to see "my fun side". After a while, she stopped saying that.

I retreated into my room, which no longer deserved to be called a study. Instead of writing, I tuned in to podcasts and news shows, casting a mist of pleasant voices I could turn up or down and which never fell silent.

As long as I could hear a voice, there was no need to be afraid.

As long as it was evening, there was no need to be afraid.

As long as she was there, there was no need to be afraid.

*

We met by chance, in a bar. Although she deigned to talk to me that first night, her eyes seldom met mine; her disinterest was almost pointed. I came straight to the point myself, asked for her number and promptly fell in love more fiercely, more unreservedly than I ever had before. In love with her looks, her resolve, her imitations of people we had just met. In love with the way she tripped over the word "millennial", and with her unremittingly high standards, which could leave me feeling pressured but also led me to believe that if I could make her happy, I couldn't possibly fail in life. For her part, she told me she had never loved a man before she met me. We went to Sicily together, our first holiday, and gave each other the same choice on a daily basis: ten more days or ten more years? A game we could afford to play, because we always knew the answer. That's one side of our story.

The other side can best be introduced by a diary entry, written shortly before we met. "There are times when I struggle to have a normal, meaningful conversation. Too downcast, too anxious etc. And I feel how this weighs on others. My one hope is that my silence goes unnoticed, that the company I'm keeping overlooks me for a while, that I disappear from view. My greatest fear is that I will end up making the person who loves me most unhappy." These episodes, when my anxiety turned to panic, tended to last a week or two, in addition to derailing occasional days scattered throughout the year. The issue wasn't so much the time consumed or a sense of unremitting darkness – there were always moments of light – it was more the unpredictability. At times, D. said, it was like bracing ourselves for a storm we couldn't see coming. Suddenly we were in the teeth of it and there was no escape.

One morning, when we had been together a month or so, D. told me she was not the nurturing kind. A chilly Sunday, low cloud, branches bare and jagged in the tree-lined square below. Her remark came out of the blue and it startled me. Had she sensed something? My answer was slow in coming: "Just as well.

I'm not the kind that needs nurturing." I hoped with all I had in me it was true.

And now, in our kitchen, I bombard her with fatalistic questions. Will I be alright? Will this ever pass? She offers the requisite understanding, but there is something mechanical about her answers.

She looks at me for a long time, and I see her struggling to say the words. She tells me she doesn't know me anymore. That I am no longer the man she fell in love with.

"But still the man you love?"

"Yes, sure. But is that enough?"

It has been a month since she took out a lease on a workspace, so we wouldn't have to spend all day at home together. In the evening, she comes back to find me in much the same state she left me in that morning. We tinker in the margins to avoid contemplating major shifts in direction.

She is wearing the red sports jersey we bought together in Berlin, denims I have seen fade with every wash. I can date and annotate each aspect of her appearance. Her tears surprise me, though I have seen them before. They follow me. Other girlfriends have cried them too. These tears are mine somehow. It's as if I am passing them on, over and over, without knowing why, without being able to stop, without shedding them myself.

She says she thinks she should move out for a while. I sink onto the steps between kitchen and living room, take deep breaths, two seconds in, three seconds out, the way I've been taught.

"It really is for the best," she says. "A chance to find myself again."

I press my palm to the floorboards, as if feeling for a heartbeat, a sign of life in this home of ours. I imagine the smell of heated wood, sawdust drifting and settling, a whiff of those first weeks when we worked on the place together. "Have you lost yourself?" I ask. "I still know where you are."

She shakes her head. Her voice softens, or perhaps her sentences have stopped getting through to me. I only grasp words in isolation: "broken", "empty", "tired".

I know the look of someone who wants to hurt me, the sound of words meant to wound – this is something else. An act of self-preservation. I tell her this is hard for me, but that she should take all the space she needs. Though I know better, I hope this concession will give her room to breathe, that my supposed generosity will work in my favour. That she will stay after all.

"You're so scared all the time," she says.

"Lots of people are scared," I reply. "All over the world."

"Perhaps it's time to find out what they're scared of. You have to do something with this, or you'll be left with nothing." There's a glimmer of compassion as her gaze holds mine. "Think of it as a journey."

"You know I hate travelling alone. People look at me funny."

"Find yourself some travelling companions."

"Will you come back?"

"I hope so. In a while."

"Ten days or ten years?"

A smile.

The end of our relationship is something I have pictured regularly. Scenes that play out in my mind, usually in the dark, when we are lying in bed. Images designed to keep harm at bay, a nip of poison to boost the immune system. The imagined ending, the final scene, the break-up, is usually a domestic affair, set in the bedroom or at an open door. Very occasionally there is a melodramatic street scene, all strained voices and wild gestures. The common theme of all these scenarios is that it's me who can't hold back the tears.

I want to say something else, something sweet, something kind, but my throat is tight. We hold each other a long time, far longer than normal, as comrades almost.

The next day her thought becomes a plan. Another day passes and she has arranged to move into the empty floor of a friend's house. I force myself to accept her choices and not protest. If I'm honest, I admire her for making a choice at all.

The morning of her departure, we agree to see each other again. In a while, when the time feels right. We are vague about when, but it will be at our favourite restaurant. She cycles off, goes to look back, then thinks better of it and stares straight ahead. I am alone. Alone but for the idea she has left me with, an idea of travel. I picture a journey to the centre of these fears of mine: their origin, their nature, where they come from, what I can learn from them, what I should do about them.

It occurs to me immediately that any exploration of my own fears has to be broader than that. If only because fear has so many meanings. There is the sudden, overwhelming, all-consuming surge we call panic. The more constant keynote of worry we know as anxiety. The highly focused fear, often triggered by one specific stimulus, which goes by the name phobia. There is social anxiety, a more amorphous fear of interacting with others. Each has its own history, has become a field of study in its own right. Fear is a response found in the smallest and the largest of creatures. But what exactly is it? An emotion, a state of being, a philosophical question, an illness? This elusive quality has always fascinated and frustrated me, knowing how real and inescapable the consequences of fear can be.

My mind starts racing. I picture travelling far and wide, in the company of characters real and fictional, philosophers and artists, patients and medics, experts and pundits, a trip through time and space. It seems to me that the paths already taken, the many studies and books already written on fear, fall short by seeking to isolate one aspect of something that is, by definition, multi-faceted and enigmatic. It's not that they're wrong, more that they're incomplete. I set myself the task of bringing these various aspects together and drawing a new roadmap along the way, one that takes in the vast scope of fear as a phenomenon. It will be a map with very few straight lines. The destination keeps shifting, as does the road itself. There will be detours and winding paths ahead, and I will no doubt meet the occasional dead end.

With routes fanning out in all directions, it is hard to work out what the first leg of this journey should be. In those first, quiet days after D.'s departure, I barely know what to do with myself. I wake up early, hours before sunrise. D. is still in the fabric of the house; the cold air is laced with her sweet Japanese perfume. I do the laundry and fold her T-shirts and socks intently, as if she were looking on. Though there is plenty of room to stretch out, I stick to my side of the bed.

Then, one morning or evening, a Monday perhaps, or a Friday, an invitation comes. From a friend who recently decided to embrace the great outdoors. He has bought a patch of land somewhere in France, with two shacks he insists on calling log cabins. He asks if I would like to visit him. The region rejoices in the name *la Vallée de Misère*. In short, it's an offer I can't refuse. I weigh myself down with two casefuls of books on fear and set off.

Halfway there, passing through Belgium, I gaze from the window of a rattling train at the ash-grey plumes above the industrial plants of Charleroi, a runaway who barely knows what he's running from. It occurs to me that this is not a beginning. Without my knowing it, this journey started long ago.

## 2

## *La Vallée de Misère*

Something inside will not let me be. This feeling hits me all the harder in my log cabin, as I gaze out at a monochrome of peaceful French pastures, unable to reconcile myself to the calm for a single second. In this vale of tears, doom-laden scenarios come thick and fast. I fret constantly, sleep in brief dreamless bouts. Shivering and confused, I cling to the one rule I have set myself: don't call her.

I know that this is not purely about D.; these feelings are older, they run much deeper. For as long as I can remember, an indefinable anxiety has been rooted in the pit of my stomach. It's there when I try to sleep and first thing when I wake up.

As it turns out, I am both one of many and an unusual case. The most reliable way to quantify someone's anxiety is to measure the level of stress hormone (cortisol) in a sample of their hair. To discover how much cortisol was buzzing around my brain, I recently submitted a hair sample to a research team at Amsterdam University Medical Centre. The average reading for someone in my part of the world is 2.7 picograms of cortisol per milligram of hair. For people with long-term mental health problems, this figure can be as high as 15 picograms.

My tests told a different story. The first, which measured my cortisol level for a three-month period, came out at 34.4, roughly thirteen times the average. Enough to raise a few eyebrows among the researchers, to put it mildly. The second test offered a month-by-month analysis: for the current month it was 74 picograms, then 87 for the previous month, 132 for the month before that and over 200 picograms for the month before that: seventy-four times the national average. This wasn't a faulty test. Out of interest, the lead researcher had also submitted a sample of her own hair to the lab. Her average came back as 0.8. The research team had never seen results like it. They speculated as to whether I might have a rare condition, a tumour that caused my glands to produce an excess of cortisol. I rejected this out of hand and, after giving it some more thought, they were inclined to agree. They then sought to reassure me: my results were so bizarre, I would probably be better off forgetting about them. Something had clearly gone wrong somewhere. "Seventy-four times higher?" I asked again. "Seventy-four," they nodded.

However bizarre the results, they didn't really change anything. The fear has always been there. My body has become attuned to it. I can be fine for a time: a keen traveller, a good friend, a loving partner. You wouldn't know there was anything wrong with me. But out of nowhere, a perceived threat – a sarcastic put down, a mixed review, some other event beyond my control – can prompt a shift in intensity. Anxiety swims into sharper focus, grows more concrete. It homes in on a single thought, a nightmarish prospect that seeps into every corner, sucks up all the air. I pass a tipping point, a critical boundary. I am in over my head.

When I am in this deep, everything I see and hear is a source of panic. I steer clear of tree-lined streets where branches block the light. No-one around me understands what is happening. I withdraw into my thoughts, my world shrinks. Time loses its familiar rhythm; clocks stop and sleep will not come. Hours are spun thin and weeks drag past, yet no one day leaves a dent on my memory. The people close to me, and even those at a cool remove, can tell at a glance. My face looks drawn, I can't sit up straight – shoulders hunched, hands tense and trembling.

Thinking and analysis are compromised when anxiety takes hold, and so it took me years to separate the perceived threat from my immediate physical reaction. The word "reaction" suggests a delay, but that is misleading: trigger and reaction occur almost simultaneously. I have often wondered if the setback that starts the chain reaction is completely arbitrary. Maybe anxiety lies dormant in my body, waiting to latch onto any pretext that comes along.

Oddly, when I am confronted with real danger, panic is sometimes conspicuous by its absence. In 2015, I was embedded as a journalist with a contingent of Dutch UN troops in Mali. In the dead of night, we were jolted awake by a series of loud, muffled blasts and the wail of a siren: an attack by Tuareg rebels. Bombs were falling around the camp: a clear and present danger that was easy to accept. I opened my tent flap and saw soldiers sprinting for safety, then calmly reached for my flip-flops and thwapped my way to the nearest shelter, brushing my teeth as I went. Perhaps this is akin to the relief some hypochondriacs feel on being handed an actual diagnosis. The danger is suddenly real, but at least you no longer need to worry that you might be losing your mind.

A similar feeling came over me at the start of the Covid pandemic. In those post-apocalyptic weeks and months, when fear and panic became a collective state of mind, I was strangely calm. I did what was expected of me and helped out where I could. A remarkable concentration asserted itself, barely even tinged with anxiety. It felt like normality inverted: as if the world had adapted to my own personal crisis mode.

The first panic attack I can remember happened when I was six or seven, at my parents' holiday cottage in the north of Holland. Near the cottage was a little stream, so dark I couldn't tell how deep the water was. A plank bridge lay across it, about one metre wide and half as long again. The wood had begun to rot and autumn leaves from the nearby forest clung to its surface. Setting foot on it one day, I heard the bridge groan and made a panicked leap for the other side. Just in time, I told myself.

The day wore on and the fear ebbed away. But that night, as I lay in bed, my heart started pounding. I found myself gagging, gasping for breath. I struggled out from under my dinosaur duvet, scrambled down from the top bunk and ran to the icy bathroom. Tears in my eyes, I caught blurred flashes of the wash-basin tap, the pale tiled walls and, behind a dingy plastic curtain, the lawnmower Mum parked in the shower to stop it rusting in the rain. She gave a worried knock on the door, then two, then three. She asked me if I was okay. I managed a few choked words of reassurance, though I had no idea what was happening to me.

Fear and fighting for breath have always been closely connected. As I started out in life, lung trouble landed me in an incubator and later in a succession of hospital beds. Asthma, croup, laryngitis – name a respiratory illness and chances are I had it. I often woke up in the middle of the night, anxious and spluttering. Mum would lead me into the bathroom and run the hot water tap until steam filled the air. Somewhere in the mist, my breath would find me again.

The strength of this connection between breathlessness and fear is also found in language. The words *angst* ("fear" in German, Danish, Swedish, Norwegian and Dutch) and *anxiety* (which has cognates in virtually all Romance languages) stem from the Indo-European root *angh*, meaning "tight" or "constricted". The Greek word *anchein*, which means "to strangle", is also derived from this root. As is the Latin *angor*, meaning "contraction" or "constriction".

In an effort to understand myself better, I have devoured accounts of fear and anxiety in recent years. Book after book, steadily filling my study. I clung to the facts they offered. Some were universal: the assertion that fear is found throughout the world. Some had a narrower focus: the cultural specifics of fear. The Indonesian and Malaysian concept of *koro*, for instance: being afraid that your genitals will shrink and eventually disappear into your lower abdomen. Or the Japanese notion of *taijin kyofusho*: the fear that your behaviour or physical presence is offensive to others. A personal favourite is the kayak anxiety experienced by the Inuit: a series of panic attacks brought on by a prolonged absence of stimuli on kayaking expeditions.

No amount of fact-finding could release me from my own fears. But I did at least discover that I am not alone.

In the darkness before dawn, I am woken by the braying of a lone donkey. The first thing I do is check my weather app. I want to know what it's like in Amsterdam, if her days are rainy or sunny. I hope for the latter; the scent of sun cream, my nose pressed to her shoulder.

The desk in my cabin – let's be honest, it's a picnic table – is strewn with articles, papers and books on fear and anxiety. There is method in my madness: the books are grouped by genre, ordered alphabetically and then chronologically – a self-made labyrinth of paper only I can negotiate. Not that anyone else would be daft enough to try.

My afternoons are spent tramping through the dense, wet woodlands, which steam ominously after a downpour. I walk until my feet are tired. The birds tuck themselves away at dusk and the hedgerows and bushes seem to sing. My friend rustles up a plate of fish fingers that somehow manage to be both charred and undercooked, after which we settle down in our deck chairs, puff on a cigar and reflect on a day that has brought nothing in particular. At the weekend, we indulge: an excursion to the pub in the nearby village, where we watch a cycle race on TV in the company of a five-toothed local in a frayed Johnny Hallyday T-shirt.

Very occasionally my friend ventures a question about D.

"Too soon" is my standard reply.

My friend's previous guest was a cousin who had multiple meltdowns and anxiety attacks in the space of a week. Wild-eyed and jittery, he hatched plans for a new start in life, plans he would never fulfil. He refused to sleep with his head to the east, and then with his head to the west. Needless to say, he wound up not sleeping at all, and was soon drinking copiously and downing pills to little or no effect. Escaping the place proved to be no mean feat either: his terror of motorways and an absolute dread of exceeding forty-five miles an hour meant it would take him the best part of a day, crawling along on country roads, to reach his home in Koblenz. Sixteen hours behind the wheel of a car, in that state! The day before I turned up, the village doctor stuck a Valium shot in his arm, which bestowed enough calm to get him through the trip.

Worldwide, an estimated 7.3 per cent of people suffer from an anxiety disorder. The label "anxiety disorder" is given on the basis of the *Diagnostic and Statistical Manual of Mental Disorders* or DSM for short, the standard manual on mental health issues which can be found in every doctor's surgery. The DSM saw the light of day in 1952, the anxiety disorder in 1980. Approximately one in five people in the Netherlands will one day develop an anxiety disorder, defined by the DSM as "excessive anxiety and worry (apprehensive expectation), occurring more days than not for at least six months, about a number of events or activities". As you read this, over one million Dutch people are experiencing these symptoms and there is no reason to assume that the situation is any different in other Western countries.

When we zoom out, the picture does not get any rosier. An estimated 18.5 million Europeans aged between 18 and 65 suffer from a phobia, and another 6.7 million from a social phobia. But the United States heads the fear rankings. One in three people in the US develop an anxiety disorder at some point in their lives. An estimated 18 per cent of the US population – some 40 million people in 2017 – are thought to be affected in any given year. That is about twice as many as are affected by depression. If these figures are starting to jangle your nerves, it may be because you suffer from arithmophobia, a fear of numbers and statistics. However, it is worth bearing in mind that these statistics and the definitions of anxiety that underpin them do not tell the whole story. For one thing, it pays to consider the interests served by the DSM and the diagnoses it contains. More of which later.

Halfway through the day, when these accounts of anxiety start to make my head spin, I leave my paper labyrinth behind and head out into the wooded valley. Passing fields dotted with huge rolls of hay, I ponder the steps that have led me here and the steps I need to take to come closer to the nature of fear, perhaps even to its core.

I come to realise that my fear of anxiety has been a key factor in every decision I have taken in life. Whatever move I make, I am careful not to rouse the monster. After all these years, it can be hard to tell where fear ends and intuition begins. There is a neurological explanation for this: registering threats alters the physiology of the brain. The release of anxiety-related hormones, such as serotonin and dopamine, makes you sharper and more alert, but also more receptive to new stimuli. Anxious people are able to perceive threats significantly faster than people with lower levels of anxiety. But this also skews how they see the world. They have an interpretation bias – a tendency to interpret benign or neutral stimuli as threatening – which is compounded by a judgement bias – an expectation that negative events will occur in the future and an assumption that the consequences of those events will be disproportionately severe. An inability to distinguish fear from intuition means that every thought, no matter how pernicious and disruptive, can feel like the truth. When you no longer know whether you can trust your intuition, you are left entirely at the mercy of your imagination in a world where one fear triggers another. Before you know where you are, anxiety has radiated outwards and infected your whole way of thinking.

It is no exaggeration to say that fear has largely shaped my interactions with others, be they friends or strangers. Friendships have been torn apart by it, relationships worn to the bone. At times I think what other people see as my character is nothing more than a system of strategies that has developed in response to my fears. Each time the monster appears, I am convinced its appearance is an admission made by my true self.

*Monster*. A word my mother used. And my grandmother and her father before her.

Returning to my cabin after another afternoon walk, I dive into Robert Louis Stevenson's 1886 novella *Strange Case of Dr. Jekyll and Mr. Hyde*. The protagonist Henry Jekyll is a medical man in Victorian London who becomes obsessed with prising apart the forces of good and evil that make up his nature. Experimenting in secret, he discovers a potion that unleashes the evil within him and his alter ego is born: the brutish Edward Hyde, a man who is entirely prey to his urges, even to the point of murder. An antidote can reverse this process but the civilised doctor slowly loses his grip on the transformation. Which of these two halves is the more tormented? Not the monstrous Hyde, in my view, but Jekyll: the man who lives in fear of the monster, dreading its resurgence and the havoc it will wreak. Dreading the next panic attack can be more suffocating than the panic itself.

In an effort to protect myself, I have often kept my life as small as possible. As a student, my main concern was evading, defusing or warding off perceived dangers. Convinced that my room had to be internet-free, I would leave my phone out in the hall. In the breaks between lectures, I took refuge in the toilets, hoping I could ride out the rising panic without anyone hearing. I developed a fondness for one particular cubicle, where a guy called René had declared his undying love for a girl called Mara by scratching a heart into the plywood.

From a rational perspective, my fears are absurd. I come from a safe and prosperous part of a safe and prosperous city in a safe and prosperous country; millions of people have it far tougher than me. I was raised by loving parents who had – and still have – my best interests at heart. Even when things have taken a turn for the worse, there has always been a safety net. I have benefited greatly from the secure, privileged circumstances of my life. They may not have been enough to shield me from fear and unhappiness, but they have ensured that I have never gone under or made irreparably bad choices. I could always count on genuine reassurance, someone to say "don't be afraid". Millions of others who struggle with fear lack access to the resources that I have been able to draw on. Where I have pulled through, many have perished, dropped out or been consigned to the margins of society.

Their place on the margins is related to the fact that, in our Western societies, fear and anxiety have become highly medicalised. (By Western societies, I basically mean Western Europe, North America, the UK and Australia.) In classical antiquity, excessive fear was predominantly seen as a physical affliction, in the Middle Ages as a sign of demonic possession, and in the nineteenth century as a philosophical problem. Today it is a mental illness, a disorder to be kept at bay with therapies and medication. But that is only the latest chapter in the story of fear.

Where does the story begin? With the Greek god Pan, a diminutive, unsightly deity whose shouting terrified both man and god, and who gives us the word *panic*? Or with Phobos – son of Ares, God of War, and Aphrodite, Goddess of Love – revered by soldiers as the personification of conflict-related fears and in whose name we recognise the word *phobia*? Or else with Nicanor and Democles, perhaps the first recorded sufferers of anxiety? Hippocrates describes Nicanor as panicking at the sound of a flute and Democles as suffering from a crippling fear of heights. "Democles [. . .] could not go along a cliff," Hippocrates wrote, "nor onto a bridge to cross a ditch of the least depth."

I riffle frantically back and forth through book after book. The cabin light burns well into the night. The hush of the valley gives me the scope to read, puzzle and ponder endlessly, while the routine of country life offers enough of a foothold to stop me losing myself among the pages. The days may drag but the weeks fly past.

And as they do, I start to feel more at ease with my subject matter, getting a grip on a force that has held me down for so much of my life. Then, on a day like any other, it occurs to me that the next chapter in this story begins with a ship and an anchor.

# 3

## Charles Darwin and the Fear within Us

On 17 September 1835, the *Beagle* dropped anchor in the pictur-esque harbour of what is now St. Stephen's Bay on San Cristóbal, a small island in the South Pacific. As soon as he went ashore, Charles Darwin was struck by the rich diversity of wildlife that surrounded him. "Little birds within 3 & four feet, quietly hopped about the Bushes & were not frightened by stones being thrown at them," he noted in his diary. "Mr King killed one with his hat & I pushed off a branch with the end of my gun a large Hawk." Darwin reasoned that these trusting creatures had known so few natural enemies that their main protective mechanism, the fear response, had not developed sufficiently. He concluded that natural selection had worked to their disadvantage, and that their lack of fear would one day drive them to extinction. Elsewhere he wrote that "even extreme fear often acts at first as a powerful stimulant".

Darwin's biological explanation of fear was in line with the simple definition already formulated by Aristotle: fear as an essential but unpleasant physical experience that is a response to imminent danger. Every organism detects and responds to danger; even a single-celled creature such as a *Paramecium* will swim away if touched with a tiny needle. Turning to ourselves, human foetuses make a movement as if to fend off danger in response to bright light. So even before we are born we exhibit behaviours that could be interpreted as fearful. The first years of our lives are not exactly free from fear either. Helpless, needy and utterly incapable of saving ourselves from harm, we crawl around surrounded by risks and dangers which we cannot understand but which still elicit a response in us. Those dangers largely lose their charge as we grow older and learn to fine-tune our fears. But sometimes the tuning goes awry. That is why Aristotle's straightforward definition is misleading. For humans, "danger" and "imminent" are diffuse concepts; some people experience more danger than others, and what one person sees as a threat might easily be shrugged off by someone else.

To understand why our experience of fear covers such a wide spectrum, it is useful to distinguish between human fear (by which I mean the kind of fear only human beings can experience) and animal fear (occurring in all animals, including humans). Roughly speaking, animal fear is a reflex and human fear is a conscious experience. Sliding my books on Darwin to one side, I open the textbooks on biology and neurology that I have lugged all the way to the valley. One thing they have in common is a keen interest in rats.

The rodent brain can be viewed as a simplified scale model of the human brain, which explains why researchers in the field of neurology tend to use mice and rats in their experiments. The rat amygdala evaluates each incoming stimulus for potential danger. When that danger seems real, the hypothalamus rapidly produces adrenaline and triggers a fight, flight or freeze response. This puts the body in crisis mode, the heightened physical state that we urbanites know from sprinting for a connecting train or arriving at the supermarket checkout only to discover we've left our wallet and phone at home. It is a mode that has its advantages. Modern research has shown that when people are slightly anxious, they perform a task more effectively than when they feel completely relaxed. Too little anxiety and your performance suffers; too much and you hit a brick wall. This is known as the Yerkes-Dodson law.

For threat detection, the amygdala, that small almond-shaped structure deep within our brain, is crucial. Remove a rat's amygdala and it becomes a stranger to fear. The same is true for humans who have sustained damage to this part of the brain. For many years, scientists at the University of Iowa have been studying a woman, known simply as SM, whose amygdala was destroyed by disease. She may well be the only person in history whom we know for certain does not experience fear. Amygdala deficiencies have also been found in psychopaths, resulting in a dramatically tempered sense of fear and an inability to recognise or understand it in others.

After being in crisis mode for a while, the rat secretes a second hormone: cortisol, the stress hormone I appear to produce in such abundance. Cortisol is needed to trigger the physical response to a threat, the actual fighting, fleeing or freezing. As the danger subsides, adrenaline levels gradually decline, until the body returns to "safe mode". Lash out at a rat and it will jump back; it flees, in other words. Keep lashing out and it will attack; it fights. But harass it long enough and it will dig itself a hole and stay there, even after you finally relent and leave it be. The cortisol has affected its brain cells and suppressed its immune system. Its fear has become chronic.

This system of physical responses is known as the fear system, although "fear detection system" would be more accurate. Once upon a time we humans, like every other species of animal, had natural enemies – lions and tigers and bears, for example – which explains why our fear detection system resembles that of a rat. Yet what I call human fear is something else: more of a layered experience than a biological reflex. As I understand it, two key differences between humans and animals have left us with a more complex relationship to fear than that of our rodent friends.

As a boy of six or seven, I went through a phase when I would lie in bed at night and obsess about my own death. For weeks, as soon as the milky light of the smiling moon on my bedside table was switched off, my thoughts would spin out of control until panic hurled me into what felt like free fall. That's how alarmed I was by the concept of death, or more precisely, by the idea that one day I would disappear completely, as if I had never existed. Schoolfriends told me their grandparents were looking down at them from heaven. I couldn't figure out how that worked. What were they sitting on? Did they chat to passing astronauts and space travellers? If so, what language did they speak? And, most important of all, what did they eat? When I asked my father how he coped with the knowledge that one day he was going to die, he replied, "I don't". It dawned on me that no grown-up ever mentioned death or gave even the slightest indication of thinking about it – a coping strategy summed up by Woody Allen's quip that he wasn't afraid of death, he just didn't want to be there when it happened. The spectre of death is always hovering; we simply choose to ignore it.

This is the first difference between animal and human fear: unlike animals, humans are aware of their finite nature from an early age. We owe this to our more highly developed limbic system, which furnishes us with emotions, and to our larger prefrontal cortex, which facilitates our capacity for language and abstract thinking. Without language, it would be impossible to conceptualise the world, to form and fathom abstractions. Other primates show many signs of self-consciousness, but what they lack is the linguistic capacity to shape abstract thoughts and ideas. We humans are the only species that lives with the absurd awareness that we will one day die. Ever since Roman poet and philosopher Lucretius pondered the nature of our being, fear of dying has been considered the primal fear from which all other human fears derive. Perhaps it's worth narrowing that down a little: death may be the prime mover but, in the end, our fears centre on our own defencelessness. And so as humans we find ourselves in the curious situation of leading more secure lives than almost any other species while also experiencing more fear. At the back of our minds, there is always the realisation that our lives are fleeting, fragile and perhaps even a little ridiculous.

Then there is the second difference. My morbid bedtime musings as a kid are just one example of what we all do on a daily basis: we use our imagination and look for words to express what we are thinking or feeling. This too is thanks to our highly developed prefrontal cortex. Grivet monkeys have a repertoire of distress signals; great tits have a specific alarm call to warn of a snake slithering in their direction. But these "languages" are concrete and limited to the here and now. What animals cannot do is formulate or convey abstractions; even the simplest form of communication about past or future events is beyond them. While the primary function of the amygdala is to register threats and produce the hormones that enable the most appropriate physical response, our prefrontal cortex is constantly engaged in interpreting our behaviour, thoughts and memories, forging them into an intelligible whole that gets us through the day. Without a prefrontal cortex, there would be no consciousness.

What does this have to do with fear?

Many studies have shown that the amygdala can respond to threatening stimuli, increasing the heart rate and activating the sweat glands, even when the test subject is unaware of the stimuli and therefore experiences no anxiety. On this basis, we can separate fear as a reflex (animal fear) from fear as an experience (human fear). Human fear is not so much characterised by the measurable physiological symptoms associated with fear; after all, a rat has those too. Rather it is distinguished by consciously experiencing those symptoms, and then seeking to understand or pinpoint the nature of that experience. What we refer to as fear or anxiety is never the unconscious animal reflex. When we use those words or think in those terms, we are classifying how we feel; we are engaging in a conscious experience.

Thanks to the uniquely human elements of our consciousness and our capacity for language, we can imagine any number of events that may or may not happen to us, from diseases that could lay us to waste, to great loves we have yet to meet or may have missed out on. Consciously or unconsciously, we are constantly simulating situations, from the possible consequences of a particular choice to an endless array of might-have-beens. We move through parallel pasts and futures, tormenting ourselves with infinite possibilities. The unsettling thing about being human is that our imagination makes it so hard to distinguish between the evils actually heading our way and the figments we fabricate for ourselves.

Night falls in the valley and rain thrums furiously on the harvester abandoned in the field. A fresh supply of books on fear is stacked in the corner of the cabin along with writings by my great-grandfather, delivered earlier in the day by a lean postman with a poignant etching for a face. On my slippers, I pad across the ice-cold floor to the window. Five cows mosey over to the straggle of trees that skirts their pasture, seeking shelter. A cloud shifts and the sky is ambushed by stars, fierce points of the palest blue. The rain settles into a steady murmur, the rafters creak. After placing the rusty percolator on the stove – another long night lies ahead – I put the neurology books away and delve into philosophy.

Fear as a disturbance of the imagination: *perturbatio imaginationis*, in the words of thirteenth-century philosopher Thomas Aquinas. In considering the relationship between fear and the imagination, Aquinas is part of a long tradition of philosophers who focus on an unlikely image: a plank.

Pondering the difference between how someone behaves when they walk across a plank that is lying on the grass – no problem – as opposed to walking across that same plank when it spans a ravine – panic stations! – Aquinas concludes that the human imagination is the main culprit when it comes to feelings of fear. Before Aquinas, the tenth-century Persian philosopher Avicenna had already observed that a person is more likely to fall when walking over a plank at a great height than when walking over a plank on the ground, though the act of walking is the same in both cases. And then there is the scholar Robert Burton, who wrote one of the first standard works on treating matters of the mind in his magnum opus *The Anatomy of Melancholy* (1621). In it, he quotes an anecdote about a Jew in France who "came by chance over a dangerous passage, or plank, that lay over a brook in the dark, without harm [and] the next day, perceiving what danger he was in, fell down dead". In other words, in the dark, without any visual input, the unfortunate man felt no fear. But in the cold light of day, seeing how easily he might have fallen, he was seized by a fear so intense that he dropped dead. Burton's conclusion: the imagination is far more powerful than reason.

Every human being has the power of imagination, and so everyone can fall prey to irrational fears. Is fear of flying (aviophobia) rational? Or only if you are a pilot? We can probably agree that some of the kids in Stephen King's *It* would have lived a good deal longer if they had demonstrated a little more coulrophobia, the supposedly irrational fear of those terrifying creatures we call clowns.

Having lived with my fears for over thirty years, the distinction between rational and irrational strikes me as largely irrelevant. Even fears that are hard to identify with can have an existential impact on the person they affect. Whether that is someone burdened with an ill-defined sense of general anxiety or someone with a phobia of nuts and bolts, ask them enough questions and you will find that they feel their very survival is at stake. Fear is always existential. And the less a fear appears to be grounded in reality, the more it says about the person: about who they are, their life story, what they want in life and what they are truly afraid of losing or missing out on. Besides, from a neurological and physiological perspective, one fear is as real as the next, whatever the trigger.

Yet, when faced with other people and their fears, we judge

them primarily on whether we see their fears as legitimate, which often comes down to how innocuous we believe the trigger to be. In everyday speech, the qualifiers "rational" and "irrational" tend to carry the subtle connotations of "justified" and "unjustified". When we regard a fear as being realistic or conceivable, we sympathise with the sufferer and offer compassion and advice. When we find their fear implausible, we mutter that they need to pull themselves together, dismiss them as an attention seeker or shun them altogether. Our experience of fear stretches back hundreds of thousands of years, yet we still talk about it in the most heavy-handed and moralistic of terms.

No-one illustrates the futility of thinking in terms of "justified" or "unjustified" fears better than Michael Bernard Loggins, a man we will meet later in this book. Born in San Francisco in 1961, Michael lives with intense anxiety and developmental disabilities that make it hard for him to accurately assess the threats he perceives. When he was encouraged to write down his fears in 1994, Michael listed 138 items, ranging from the medical, the paranoid and the abstract to remarkably specific fears, such as his favourite noodles being eaten by a guy called Douglas. He circulated his lists in the form of hand-stapled mimeographs, which were later collected and published in a small, printed edition. Michael Bernard Loggins demonstrates something my instinct has always told me: that the fear of dying needn't be taken more seriously than the fear of Douglas scoffing your favourite snack. In fact, noodle deprivation can be more immediate and overwhelming than the absolute inevitability of death.

How does it feel when fear strikes? The outward signs can be summed up by the sensations I felt as a boy, gasping and teary-eyed in the bathroom of my parents' holiday cottage: you sweat, your heart races, your chest tightens, your muscles tense, your mouth goes dry, your fingers tingle and your stomach churns. The sheer physicality of this experience is a crucial aspect of what fear is. This is underlined by the American philosopher William James, often credited as the "father of psychology", who wrote in 1890: "What kind of an emotion of fear would be left if the feeling neither of quickened heart-beats nor of shallow breathing, neither of trembling lips nor of weakened limbs, neither of goose-flesh nor of visceral stirrings, were present, it is quite impossible for me to think. Can one fancy the state of rage and picture no ebullition in the chest, no flushing of the face, no dilatation of the nostrils, no clenching of the teeth, no impulse to vigorous action, but in their stead limp muscles, calm breathing, and a placid face?"

But even if, in this state of constricted consciousness, you were able to pick apart the various faltering physiological processes, even if you could quantify each hormone your brain produces when you feel threatened, still the exact nature of your fear would elude you. It's not your tears that make you cry, not your vomit that makes you nauseous. The conscious experience of fear, how it is perceived – by definition a subjective process – is an essential element of fear itself.

The perception of fear has traditionally been the domain of philosophers. The fact that you never know exactly where your fear comes from prompted Martin Heidegger to argue that fear is nowhere in particular: "Therefore that which threatens cannot bring itself close from a definite direction within what is close by; it is already 'there', and yet nowhere; it is so close that it is oppressive and stifles one's breath, and yet it is nowhere." Fear is the aggressor; you are passive. And yet fear comes from within. Are you responsible for your fears, or do your fears absolve you of all responsibility? Are you perpetrator or victim? Can you be both at the same time?

The immersive nature of fear as an experience is found in almost all descriptions by those who have been through it. The most poetic and at the same time the most recognisable description I have come across is from a dissertation on fear and anxiety disorders, written by Dutch psychiatrist Gerrit Glas. In it, he quotes a thirty-five-year-old man identified only by the initial B., who was hospitalised for psychiatric care on several occasions. B. described his anxiety as "An empty feeling in the stomach, which moves and can be felt. It is both a feeling and a physical sensation, in your head and in your body. It is a single whole, and it's almost impossible to work out exactly where it starts." The ferocity of panic, the extent to which fear can seize you by the throat, overwhelming you until you see no way out: there is no real way to quantify or demonstrate all this but I can attest to it, as can countless others. Perhaps you can too.

Charles Darwin, who wrote so lucidly about fear as a biological phenomenon, suffered from debilitating breakdowns, palpitations and frequently recurring episodes of hyperventilation. At times, he was housebound, barely able to work and vomited several times a day. A comprehensive study of Darwin's diaries, letters and documented medical history, conducted several years ago, led doctors in the United States to conclude that by today's standards Darwin would undoubtedly have been diagnosed with a panic disorder. Four symptoms out of thirteen provide sufficient basis for such a diagnosis; Darwin had nine of them. Anyone on the right side of the line between good health and ill health could find that they have crossed it tomorrow; how and where that line is drawn is something I will return to in later chapters.

I snap the last book shut. Having committed the fundamentals to paper, it feels like my stay in the Vallée de Misère is reaching its natural conclusion. It's time to leave the written word behind for a while and dig deeper into my own fears, which may not be entirely my own after all. It occurs to me that members of my family have experienced similar symptoms and that anxiety might have been running through our genes for centuries. Or is that putting too much faith in biology? Should I be examining the circumstances of their lives instead? In any case, I have an inkling as to where, and in whose company, I should begin. The place: Indonesia. The person: Jaap Kunst, my great-grandfather.

After booking my ticket, I email a number of experts whose work in recent years has focused on fear and anxiety. Their insightful contributions will pop up from time to time along the way. I tuck a number of key works into my suitcase or save them on my laptop, and ask my friend to send the rest on to my home address. In a field the colour of rust, knee-deep in grass and thistles, I find a spot where the internet connection is least feeble and download the maps I expect to need in Indonesia. Trudging back to the cabin, I wonder whether I should think of fear less as a monster and more as a navigator beside me in the car, albeit one who refuses to share the road map. He may switch places during this trip, take a back seat for a while or hide himself away in the boot. At times he might elbow his way into the driver's seat, but the fact that you are reading this means he did not manage to stay there long.

My final evening in France arrives and my friend and I share a stoic last supper of fish fingers washed down with Carrefour wine. Before the clock strikes eleven, we give each other a brotherly hug and, for fear sentimentality might get the better of us, keep our thoughts to ourselves. I'm relieved to be departing without a shot of Valium.

In bed, my thoughts drift back to the plank bridge of my boyhood holidays. I follow Avicenna's template and imagine it spanning a ravine rather than a small stream in the tame Dutch countryside. Instead of crossing in fear, I gaze calmly into the depths. Danish philosopher Søren Kierkegaard likened fear to an abyss and wrote that "to know anxiety is an adventure which every man has to affront". I walk on until I find myself in the Far East. Jakarta to be precise.

# 4

## The Spell of the Gamelan

It is a hot, sticky day in Jakarta, and the acrid smell of Pertamax petrol lingers in the streets. From the vantage point of this tower by the harbour, I picture their ship disappearing over the horizon: Jaap Kunst, his wife Katy and their three children – family from three generations ago.

After fourteen years in Indonesia – or the East Indies as they knew it – they sailed for the Netherlands in March 1934 aboard the *Sibajak*, an ocean liner operated by Royal Rotterdam Lloyd, one of the largest and most opulent to make the voyage to the Dutch colony. On that return journey, Jaap reports feeling wretched. He would burst into tears for no reason, clutching the railing as he battled "what German psychiatrists refer to as *frei flottierende Ängste*". Free-floating fears. As I look back at my family history, the diary kept by Jaap Kunst, my great-grandfather, presents me with the earliest traces of fear. From Jaap, the trail leads through my grandmother to my mother and on to me. This string of lives is relevant because it may shed light on the degree to which genetic predisposition plays a role in the transmission of fear. What was the source of the *Ängste* that plagued Jaap on board the *Sibajak*? To find out, we need to go back a little further: to 1919, when Jaap arrived in the Indies. Not chasing fortune or adventure, but on a quest for music.

*

Born in the northern Dutch city of Groningen in 1891, Jacob Kunst – Jaap to his family and friends – was, in his own words, saddled with the "hereditary defect" of music. Jaap had a phonographic memory and could read notes before he could write. At the age of three, he heard his father play a curious melody, which he memorised from start to finish and recognised instantly when it was played at a cello recital half a century later, never having heard it in the intervening years. Aged four, Jaap threw a birthday tantrum when he unwrapped his present to find a toy violin instead of a real one. He had to wait another two years for his first proper instrument, the one he would play until the day he died.

Jaap's school record was far from exemplary, something he put down to "inner tensions". When the First World War broke out in 1914, he was quick to sign up as a home guard volunteer. Unfortunately, in the neutral Netherlands, the only weapon he was allowed to wield was a gun that popped a cork to scare off dogs. To make matters worse, every training exercise ground to a premature halt at the local pub due to the lieutenant's "chronic thirst". As soon as the armistice was signed in 1918 and the seas were free again, Jaap began making plans for an ambitious voyage. Teaming up with a pianist and a *diseuse lyrique* – the spoken word artists of their day – he formed a musical trio, with himself in the twin roles of violinist and animal impressionist. On borrowed money, they set sail from Rotterdam in 1919. The plan was to recoup their outlay with the revenue generated by performances in the Indies, an optimistic scheme that soon succeeded. Jaap fell under the spell of the Indonesian archipelago, and when the other members of the trio returned to the Netherlands in May 1920, Jaap stayed on. His reasons were twofold.

On Christmas Eve 1919, while visiting the Sultan of Yogyakarta, he had been introduced to the Javanese gamelan, a type of music he described in a letter to his mother as "sacred", "centuries old" and "overwhelming". Jaap resolved there and then to "unlock the gamelan's secrets". He had found something that gave his life direction, an impetus that tempered his inner tensions. In the years that followed, whenever his civil service job allowed, he would travel the length and breadth of Java to record its musical culture. Part explorer, part curator, he did for Indonesia's musical traditions what Alan Lomax would later do for folk music in Europe and the United States. Jaap Kunst, the Netherlands' first ethnomusicologist, became world-famous in the smallest of circles.

His second reason for staying on in the Indies was even more poetic. If family lore is to be believed, he met the love of his life, Katy van Wely, during one of his performances, most likely at the court of Paku Alam VII, a prince from Yogyakarta. "Beautiful Katy" was the daughter of a high-ranking official of mixed descent, whose greatest fear was that his children would end up "going native".

Before long, Jaap and Katy began to write to each other. In his first letter, dated April 1921, Jaap invited Katy to confide in him, if she so wished, whenever she was feeling out of sorts. "I believe I have the capacity to understand practically anything a person might have to endure in terms of conflict and inner misery," he assured her. In his fifth letter, he went into greater detail about the emotional turmoil he regularly suffered. "In the morning, my old enemy reared its head once again: that wretched restlessness, not to say fear, which thus far has been the perpetual companion to every overture I have made to another person. Shyness, a lack of psychological resilience, constriction of consciousness: I do not know what it is, but at several points in my life it has caused me to think: if only I were dead, for it has brought others and myself such unhappiness at times." But through Katy, he thought this might change. "Oh, if you, who are such a delight to me," he wrote in the same letter, "with whom I feel such a close inner bond, if you who understand me so well [. . .] could give me the same affection and friendship that I, with all my heart, wish to give you, if you were able and willing to help overcome this imbalance, this psychological deficit in me, then I might become a different person and welcome the prospect of a new life." A warning, a plea and a love letter all in one. Jaap's words struck a chord with Katy; she had never met such a sensitive man. They did not become friends. That same year, on 4 October 1921, they married amid a sea of flowers. As yet, there was no sign of anxiety; that is to say, love was stronger.

Not long after their wedding, Jaap and Katy moved to the city of Bandung, a lush mountain setting where the climate was relatively cool and dry. Bandung had a closed sewer system and this minimised the spread of infectious diseases such as typhoid and dysentery. Photographs from the time show pristine streets lined with newly built white houses. The people cycling past could be figures in a life-size architect's model. On 11 August 1922, Katy gave birth to their first child: Sjuwke, my grandmother. In her baby book, Jaap writes, "Since day one she has reacted to sounds: whistling stops her crying. Could she be musical? Her tiny hands, with their long nimble fingers." Describing Sjuwke at the age of one, he notes in a letter, "Our daughter takes a great interest in musical instruments." Jaap observed that the Besuki angklung, a traditional thirteenth-century musical instrument made of bamboo tubes, made her especially happy. Katy had a rather different take on their daughter's predilections: "She still finds music extremely unpleasant and it brings on desperate crying fits. She has learned to tolerate singing, but the violin is an instrument of torment." The violin, of all things.

A few days after my visit to Jakarta – most of which was spent warding off mosquitoes and trying to stop copies of my great-grandfather's letters from going limp in the heat – I become a figure in the architect's model and walk the streets of Bandung, the city where Jaap's family experienced the best of times, but where he also endured many fears. His old enemy had stalked him to the mountains of Java and was waiting for its chance; as soon as Jaap had too much on his mind, it would strike.

Reaching into my bag, I pull out a photocopied image of Jaap. I stare at it for a time, hoping to see my features in his, but his cheekbones are too sharp, his face too narrow. It's been a long day. I lost my way, gawped blankly at street signs, soldiered on and got even more lost. Eventually, my brain creaked into gear and I was able to forge connections between my street plan and the historical sources. After Indonesia gained its independence, almost every street name was changed, transforming the entire city into a *roman à clef.*

The Kunsts lived in three different houses in Bandung, two of which are still standing. One is now home to a vague privacy firm and has been remodelled to the hilt; the original building at its core is barely identifiable. The other building, more of a glorified shack, currently houses a nail salon which offers customers the option of a "vagina spa", number 14 on the menu. The third building was demolished to make way for a colossal white bank. The privacy firm's headquarters was where fear entered the family's life. It was there that Katy first witnessed one of Jaap's "episodes", which according to their daughter Sjuwke became more or less an annual occurrence. They always followed the same pattern, beginning with a phase during which Jaap worked extremely hard, almost to the point of mania, and would tolerate no interruptions. Then came the collapse. "He would sit motionless in a chair for days at a time," Sjuwke recalls. "He wouldn't lift a finger for us, not for me, not for Mammi. Then, one day he would get up, strap his violin to his back and leave the house without saying where he was going. It later turned out that he went to see friends, to make music. After a few weeks, he would call and timidly ask Mammi if she felt like coming over. She always went. It was the sign that he was back. That he was hers again."

Time and again, it was Katy who helped him get back on his feet. Through almost forty years of marriage, she ran the household and supported Jaap in his research. Little was said about his breakdowns and it never occurred to anyone to send for a doctor. The common view was that his "sensitivity" was part of his genius: he was highly strung, a special case. "People thought his bouts of depression were ever so interesting," Sjuwke remembers. As soon as he was back to his old self, Jaap threw himself into his research once again. That meant fieldwork: with his trusty Edison Amberola Model 50, an ultramodern phonograph of the day, he made countless musical recordings on wax cylinders. These were later shipped to Berlin, where moulds were made that enabled the recordings to be duplicated. Jaap combed the countryside, mostly on horseback with the heavy Edison in tow, through jungles and over dirt roads, paying local singers in cigarettes and hand mirrors, anything to coax them to perform. Wherever he went, Jaap purchased musical instruments, which he brought home as prized possessions or took to the archive in Batavia (present-day Jakarta), where Katy catalogued them. Every last cent was ploughed into his research, which he pursued with the zeal of a religious mission. He describes this best in a letter from November 1923, in which he talks about an "irrational obedience to the inner urge that propels me along the path set out by my inclination and disposition".

In letters to friends and colleagues, my great-grandfather attributed his breakdowns to external factors, the practicalities of life. In May 1922, he wrote of the dire financial straits in which the family found themselves as a "time of malaise". In September of that year, he mentioned problems arising from "the combination of gamelan research, the birth of the baby, paying eighteen months' worth of back taxes, moving home and refurbishing". Even so, they were "making the best of things". He regularly defaulted on his bills, as evidenced by dozens of written apologies. On 18 February 1924, Katy and Jaap welcomed their second child into the world, a son they christened Jacobus, Japie for short. Two years later, on 2 January 1926, the family was rounded out with the arrival of another son, Egbert Diederik. A growing family, holding down a job, their ever-expanding research, constant money worries – all this began to wear Katy and Jaap down. Exhaustion loomed and fear crept through the house.

In letters from October 1926, Jaap spoke of "an indisposition due to over-tiredness" and even "a recurring state of being almost overworked". Things didn't improve. "The uncertainty – for so long now – is crippling for my peace of mind and keeps me awake at night," he wrote in September 1928. When the stock markets crashed in 1929, ushering in a global economic depression, life for the Kunsts became harder still. Yet by 1931, the family home contained 237 wax cylinders and 245 instruments. Only once does Jaap stop short of blaming his worries entirely on external factors. In a letter to a historian friend Johan Huizinga, he wrote in 1932, "I must take care not to work myself too hard [. . .] The medicine man says my nervous system has taken a bit of a drubbing." I've reread this passage several times. The nervous system: for him, that was the key.

If he had consulted a European doctor rather than a medicine man, Jaap would probably have been diagnosed with neurasthenia, a condition associated with nervous debility. Referred to as "the English malady", this nervous condition was seen as an affliction of the upper classes or captains of industry and commerce in eighteenth-century Britain. It would be the nineteenth century before the rest of the Western world started using the label, as people became captivated by modernity in all its innovative and unsettling guises: the railways, the telephone, urbanisation, photography. People whose sensibilities failed to absorb these shocks to the system were seen as suffering from neurasthenia.

The first use of "neurasthenia" as a psychopathological term was by US psychiatrist E.H. Van Deusen, who, after doing his rounds at the Kalamazoo institution where he worked, noted that a new "form of nervous prostration" had emerged, "a disorder of the nervous system" caused among other things by "excessive mental labour, especially when conjoined with anxiety". George

Miller Beard, the first successful American author in the field of psychiatry, popularised the term in 1869. The condition, jokingly referred to as "Americanitis", covered a multitude of symptoms: general malaise, headaches, dilated pupils, dizziness, tinnitus, numbness, nausea, flushed cheeks, insomnia, alcoholism or drug addiction, chills, hysteria, lassitude, irritability, anxiety, compulsive thoughts and sexual dysfunction. Neurasthenia is often seen as the nineteenth-century equivalent of what we would now call a burnout. But fear, anxiety and phobias, not regarded as separate categories at the time, were central to the clinical profile from the outset. In the period before neurasthenia became commonly diagnosed, some doctors and scientists had advocated looking at fear as a separate issue, but their tendency to focus on its physical symptoms, such as dizziness and breathlessness, meant that their reports were usually published in medical rather than psychiatric textbooks. Less acute and physical forms of fear, what we now call anxiety, were mostly regarded as normal, everyday afflictions.

No consensus emerged on the source of an overactive fear response. In the mid-nineteenth century, the influential Hungarian ear, nose and throat specialist Maurice Krishaber believed that excessive fear was caused by unstable blood corpuscles. A contemporary of Krishaber's, the Hungarian-Austrian physician Moriz Benedikt, thought that pathological changes in the ear were the main cause of panic attacks. But theories that viewed chronic fears primarily as a physical ailment eventually lost out to those put forward by neurologist and founder of psychoanalysis Sigmund Freud. In 1894, Freud called for a new category to be established within neurasthenia: anxiety neurosis. Freud's call was widely heeded and his idea met with next to no criticism. No-one was more surprised by this than Freud himself, since – as he observed – he had "adduced hardly any examples and quoted no statistics".

The terms "neurasthenia" and "anxiety neurosis" are nowhere to be found in Jaap's letters. The same is true of "melancholy", a popular term at the time and one with a long history that warrants a brief excursion into antiquity and the work of Hippocrates of Kos, who lived from 460 to 370 BCE. Central to Hippocrates' highly influential teachings was the notion that our health depends on the balance between four distinct fluids or humours in the human body: phlegm, blood, yellow bile and black bile. A perfect mixing ratio (*krasis*) of these humours was thought to produce an ideal, harmonious state of being. An excess of phlegm would manifest itself as an overly calm and unruffled temperament, the root of our word "phlegmatic". A surplus of black bile, however, would spawn a mood that was gloomy or maudlin: the Greek *melan-* (black, dark) combining with *cholē* (bile) to give us the word "melancholy".

With the odd tweak, Hippocrates' teachings stood their ground well into the Middle Ages, only invalidated when the anatomical experiments of scientists in the sixteenth and seventeenth centuries led to a more accurate understanding of the workings of the human body. By then, the term "melancholy" had taken on a life of its own, and in Jaap's time it had gone from being a phenomenon associated with bodily fluids to a broader precursor of what we now call depression. Melancholy pinned you to the ground and darkened your mood. But the term also covered a variety of symptoms we now associate with other psychiatric conditions, such as anxiety disorder, obsessive-compulsive disorder and delusional behaviour. By the eighteenth century, fear was accounting for an ever larger part of the catch-all condition of "melancholy", to the extent that leading French physician J.F. Dufour viewed "fear and sadness" as its main symptoms. Some doctors even deployed fear to bring on melancholy, a way of counterbalancing excessively passionate and impulsive behaviour: "Fear being a passion that diminishes excitement, may therefore be opposed to the excesses of it, and particularly to the angry and irascible excitement of maniacs," William Cullen, personal physician to philosopher David Hume, wrote in 1785. Red-hot pokers could be a particularly effective way of upping anxiety levels, it was suggested.

There's another aspect of melancholy which strikes me as

relevant to Jaap's case: the fact that, unlike depression today, it was widely accepted among learned, creative and intellectual men as an unfortunate side effect of their tendency towards contemplation, and had been since the time of Aristotle. The total absence of the word "melancholy" from Jaap's letters and his children's recollections suggests to me that he had huge difficulty admitting that his problems not only stemmed from the circumstances of his life on Java – the island was on the brink of economic collapse at the time – but were also a deep-seated part of his make-up. Only in his early letters to Katy did he seem able to be completely honest.

In 1930, there was a glimmer of hope: Jaap's calling and his working life dovetailed miraculously when he was given the post of government musicologist. The family moved again, within Bandung. The local community lent a hand and the open-topped wagon transporting his collection of instruments became "an orchestra on wheels, rolling along in the sunshine". This new position meant that Jaap was on the road more than ever, while Katy stayed at home with the children. He trekked through the jungle, crossed rickety bamboo bridges and witnessed celebrations in wild places where men and women danced in their traditional finery: white plumes, red and white beads, a feathered staff, quiver and bow, wearing "bells around the ankles and on their derrière". As long as he was on the move, his fears could not overtake him.

But December 1931 dealt a crushing blow. The funding for Jaap's musicological endeavours dried up. He was assigned "some legal position or other", work that did not interest him in the slightest. To a friend he wrote that "these sudden changes and the prospect of once again having to perform desperately tedious administrative work weighs heavily on my mind [. . .] The discontinuation of this research is enough to drive a man to tears." Katy's health also began to fail; she lost weight. The children were sickly. Enough was enough: plans for their return to the Netherlands were set in motion. By this time, they were sharing their home with almost twelve hundred instruments.

"I am curious as to whether I shall set eyes upon the Indies again this year," he wrote on the eve of his departure in 1934, "or indeed whether I shall return to Java at all. For several reasons, it is more desirable for me to try to build a new life in Europe. Neither I nor my wife fare well in this climate; and I still feel that my nervous system has suffered as a result of the hard work." Jaap's words proved prophetic. He would never see Java again.

*

I spend three weeks in my great-grandfather's company, mulling over words and impressions from a life I had always left unexamined, a life that foreshadows my own. Then it's time for me to pack my bags too. On my last day in Bandung, I attend an evening of traditional Javanese music, a celebration of the gamelan and the angklung, the instrument to which Jaap was convinced my grandmother had taken a liking at the age of one. The sound is warm and inviting, rich in resonance and reverb; a harmonic cacophony that makes sense as long as you hear it and slips from your grasp the second it stops. Perhaps that's what drew Jaap Kunst to Javanese music in the first place: its enigmatic nature, the way it resists analysis. A spell that enthrals you as you listen, that draws you into a space outside yourself for a time. Instead of a ticket, tonight's listeners have each been given a miniature angklung on a chain to hang around their neck. On an impulse, I pocket it rather than handing it back on my way out – a fragile, illicit memento of a man I feel I know, but never met.

*

As we know, Jaap's voyage back to the Netherlands was something of an ordeal. First, there was the disappearance of little Japie.

49

When the ship left port after docking in Colombo, Sri Lanka, he was nowhere to be found. After a frantic search he was discovered hiding in a corner in the engine room, transfixed by the pumping of the giant pistons. The other disruptions centred on Jaap's emotional state: his sudden fits of crying, his need to cling to the railing, his free-floating fears. Before the voyage was even over, he began to fantasise about a return to the Indies, in a while, when everyone was fit to travel again. The Kunsts disembarked in Rotterdam, the main port of what was to be their homeland from that day on: they were Hollanders once more.

After a year in the Netherlands, Jaap's doctor warned him never to set foot in the tropics again, let alone inflict such a journey on his wife and children. He resigned himself to this fate in the hope that staying put would finally rid him of his "wretched insomnia". It didn't. Reacclimatising to Dutch society proved gruelling. Money was scarce, interest in his life's work even more so. Every trip abroad only served to remind him of what he had left behind on Java: the freedom, the wide-open spaces and, most of all, the music – the spell cast by the gamelan. Around 1939, against doctor's orders, he began to make detailed plans to sail for the Indies, as soon as the family were back on their feet. In May 1940, they were all set. The necessary purchases had been made, their luggage had been sent ahead and had already reached Genoa. And then on 10 May, war broke out. Their ship would never sail. Their suitcases turned up in the Netherlands months later, scuffed and battered.

In the misery of the Nazi-occupied Netherlands, music was Jaap's only comfort. During the last winter of the war, when fuel and power supplies ran out and much of the population went hungry, Jaap regularly got together with his friends. "When we played, we barely noticed everything else," he wrote. Musicians and listeners alike would bring along a stick of wood or a few lumps of peat to warm the numbness from the players' fingers so that they could produce music worth listening to. But as the war drew to a close, Jaap's fears did not relent. His breakdowns became increasingly frequent and even harder to live with now there were no identifiable work-related or war-related causes, and no appreciative souls around to attribute the condition to his genius. In the 1950s, Jaap travelled the world when he could, giving lectures. Everywhere he went, he played the violin. Very occasionally he managed to find himself a "good Indies breakfast" of coffee, pisang, papaya, bread and canned butter.

By 1956, his travelling days were just about over and the time had come to write his memoirs. Only then, with the end in sight, did he dare to open up about the "inner tensions" that had dogged him as a schoolboy, about the fears that beset him on his ocean voyage back to the Netherlands, about the unspecified "anxiety-fuelled catastrophes" that had put paid to his engagements until he met Katy. "A residue of that fear," he wrote, "in the form of a recurring yet fickle heaviness of heart prevents me from enjoying life in perfect harmony." It was thanks to his "sweet and sensible" wife that he had been able to function, a woman who understood the "abnormality" in his "inner structure", the woman who spared and saved him. Jaap died on 7 December, 1960, a cold, grey day in a bitter Dutch winter. He left behind a correspondence of 8,500 letters, shelves of scholarly books, folders and notebooks, endless telegrams about his lack of money and crates full of photographs of musical instruments. Every ridge in the wood, every crack in the varnish had been recorded and meticulously indexed. The photographs now reside in the cooled depot of an Amsterdam museum collection. A life's work becomes a catalogue, a human life a resource.

\*

Of Jaap's three children, I only know Sjuwke, my grandmother, the infant angklung player. To this day, a deep kinship exists between us. When I visit her at the nursing home, one look is often enough. This bond is intimately connected with our shared experience of fear, as if we are in on the same secret. In Sjuwke, Jaap's fears from the Indies became a Dutch story.

Sjuwke takes after her father in that she has always had a strong "inner urge". Jaap noted that, even as a little girl, she declared that she could draw "remarkably well". In the Netherlands of the 1930s, her education took her from the village school on the small island of Terschelling to an all-girls secondary in Arnhem and on to a Montessori grammar school in Leusden. By her own account, she was a steady, diligent girl who sketched and drew at every opportunity. This interest led her to visit an artists' colony in the southern province of Limburg. The months she spent there, at a castle in the country, may well have been her happiest ever, enough to fuel a lifetime of longing. While German forces occupied the Netherlands and the freight trains rumbled eastwards, she swam every day in the cool, clear waters of the Meuse, cycled over the rolling hills and sketched forests, trees, roads, water. Occasionally she would catch the eye of a young man, but she shrugged off their advances.

This changed in 1941 when she met my grandfather Geurt outside Amersfoort railway station. Not that they were strangers; she had long been friends with his sister. But running into him at the station, she suddenly found herself admiring a man as mature as he was handsome. Geurt had just returned from Rome, where – as a novice artist bowled over by the churches and the age-old traditions – he had converted to Catholicism. Later he described their encounter: "I had travelled for days in a blacked-out train. My homeland was bitterly cold and I dragged my suitcase across the frozen snow. The first familiar face I saw belonged to Sjuwke Kunst, one of my sister Else's classmates, who was cycling in my direction but did not wave back at me." Sjuwke had her reasons: the sight of Geurt standing there with his heavy suitcase made her painfully aware of her runny nose and the tatty cloth she was wearing by way of a headscarf to keep off the worst of the cold. Mortified that he might see her in such a state, she sped past him. It was an anecdote they both dished up with pride: Geurt because he had finally conquered her, Sjuwke because she had been worth the chase.

Geurt and Sjuwke moved in together. Home was a narrow, draughty house on Lijnbaansgracht in Amsterdam. Times were hard. Geurt was a medal maker, Sjuwke a draughtswoman and sculptor, not skills that were in great demand in wartime – or at any time, come to that. They had four children: a son and three daughters. My mother, the third child, was born in 1949.

The war was over, but sorrow and scarcity cast a veil over the time that followed. Almost one million Dutch people owned little more than the clothes on their backs; my grandparents were no exception. They struggled to make ends meet. Sjuwke was not ashamed to use old rags and cloths to make the children's clothes. Sometimes, when she felt the walls closing in on her and when there was not enough food, Sjuwke would take the children and stay with her mother for a while. Jaap's widow, his beautiful Katy, lived alone in a house crammed with Indonesian totems and dusty memorabilia.

Post-war life took a heavy toll on my grandmother. She suffered intermittent breakdowns that could last months. It's still not easy for her to talk about these episodes. "I'm a sponge. I absorb tension," she says. "I have a sensitive nervous system, just like my father." She describes her ordeal in terms of exhaustion. "I was living at my limits. The stress and the strain, there was no end to it. And suddenly everything was out of control. It was like a mental ambush. It knocked me off balance. And on top of that there was the feeling of letting everyone down, that you can't do anything right, you and your thick head." It was many years before she felt able to talk to me about these experiences, the times when "it" threatened to take hold again. It began with an increasing sense of unease and agitation, accompanied by relentless worries and fears. "It rushed at you, pounced on you. There was no fighting it." She felt smothered, trapped. Unable to sleep, she battled her way through till morning. The next day, she lived in fear of nightfall, afraid to go to bed. She knew losing another night's sleep would leave her weaker. It became harder to stand her ground. Fear of not sleeping kept her wide awake. Until, in the end, she hardly slept at all.

This was not lost on her children. "When we came home from school, we knew right away," my mother recalls. "The way she sat at the table, her voice unsteady, eyes drifting around the room, something desperate in her gaze. All at once she was incapable of doing anything, utterly drained. The simplest chore became too much, every thought was unsettling. Words of comfort were lost on her. Her grip on the order of things, her connection to others kept slipping. There were moments when things seemed to get through to her – how much we loved her, that this would soon pass – but they washed away as soon as we stopped talking. Nothing we said stuck. It was scary, as if she was possessed by some dark force."

These episodes came and went, leaving their mark on the young family. Solid and pragmatic, Geurt did his best to be a kind and loving husband, but he barely understood what was happening. The children certainly didn't: unable to tally their behaviour with their mother's mood, they were helpless. At times, they did wonder: are we to blame? My aunt Clara remembers her mother seeking comfort, snuggling up to her in bed in search of solace. Perhaps it *was* their fault: hadn't Mamma told them she was happiest when she was drawing?

Something was out there, something that would hide for months, then strike suddenly and transform their sweet, caring mother into a frightened, doleful spectre; something that broke her in half, into two halves, two people who were nothing alike. As a little girl, this entity seemed like a monster to my mother. "And then, as suddenly as it had appeared, it vanished," she says. "Gone were the fear and chaos. Her voice became firmer, her gaze less panicky. The light came back, there was room to breathe. It left as quickly as it had come, for no apparent reason, and she refused to be reminded of it. My mother has always had two faces."

*

Is there more to be said about that "something" at the root of this division within my grandmother? The venerable label of "melancholic" was never intended for women, who had to make do with the subcategory of "uterine melancholy", otherwise known as hysteria (derived from *hystéra*, the Greek for "womb"). In essence, hysteria amounted to the same thing as melancholy, only shorn of the positive connotations of genius and special status. The notion that the womb or uterus could move of its own accord and negatively impact a woman's mental health existed as far back as Ancient Egypt (1900 BCE). One of the earliest medical documents, the Ebers Papyrus, which dates from about 1600 BCE, describes the main symptom of this uterine ailment as a suffocating sensation. The Ancient Egyptian solution was to nudge the womb back into its "natural position", sometimes after smearing a caustic, pungent substance around the vulva. Hippocrates was the first to use the term "hysteria". Because the womb was restless and prone to wander, he argued, a woman's inner balance was vulnerable to disturbance. He reasoned that the female body was cold and wet, and therefore at risk of rotting, a process that could bring on anxiety, tremors and the aforementioned feeling of suffocation. According to Hippocrates, it took sex with a man to "cleanse" a woman's body. Only in the seventeenth century, thanks to the work of Oxford scholar Thomas Willis and French doctor Charles Le Pois (who equated hysteria with hypochondria) did it become widely recognised that the condition known as hysteria had nothing whatsoever to do with the womb.

By Sjuwke's time, the terms "melancholy" and "uterine melancholy" were losing their scientific clout. Another label had emerged, a new name for an old disease: "depression", derived from the Latin *deprimere*, meaning "to press down" or "to lower".

As far back as 1860, the word "depression" had begun to crop up in medical dictionaries to describe the state of being downcast or in low spirits. Historians believe it was this element – the "down" in downcast, the "low" in low spirits – that prompted the rise of this new medical term. Melancholy not only came to be seen as too broad, but also as failing to capture the cheerless, despondent state that doctors observed in their patients. It therefore broke up into a number of syndromes, the main one being depression. The first edition of the authoritative *Régis Practical Manual of Mental Medicine*, published in 1885, defined depression as "the opposite condition to excitement", characterised in extreme cases by "an absolute immobility or stupor". Physician Sir William Gull, who coined the term anorexia nervosa, wrote of mental depression "occurring without apparently adequate cause". In the early twentieth century, with psychiatry gaining ground as a field of medicine in its own right, "melancholy" lost out to the more precise and scientific-sounding concept of "depression" once and for all. Freud went on to explore the relationship between grief and melancholy but increasingly it came to be used as a vaguely descriptive term, while depression entered the medical lexicon.

My grandmother Sjuwke also found herself faced with this relatively new label, much to her annoyance. "The doctor called it depression . . . a fat lot of good that did. He sent me to a psychiatrist; that didn't work either. What a moaning Minnie he was. No use whatsoever." The thought of taking medication for this condition horrified her. She did undergo a course of sleep therapy, a method developed by Swiss psychiatrist Jakob Klaesi, in which the patient was sedated and slept eighteen to twenty hours a day for a two-week period. This was supposed to bring rest, but all it did was knock Sjuwke for six. She eventually tried sleeping pills, then antidepressants. "A chemical disruption, like being poisoned." To this day, she views paracetamol with suspicion.

Now, at the age of ninety-six, she still suffers occasional breakdowns, but the troughs are far less deep. At the nursing home where she lives, she lies low and waits for her depression to pass, listening to classical music on the radio. Pianos and clarinets are especially soothing. And it turns out she's got nothing against the violin after all.

*

Can Sjuwke's anxiety and breakdowns be accounted for by a stifling lack of self-fulfilment, her artistic talent suppressed in favour
of raising a family, her desires subordinated as a matter of course
to those of the paterfamilias, the patriarch? It's a question that my
mother – the third of Sjuwke's four children – regularly asked herself. Self-fulfilment, subordination: terms from another time, from
the 1960s, when the tight-lipped stoicism of post-war reconstruction
gave way to free expression and feminism, and greater attention was
paid to the individual psyche, the true self, the stirrings of the soul.

My mother studied at the University of Amsterdam, a warren
of buildings in the heart of the old city. Her reason for enrolling
was much the same as my own when I followed in her footsteps
over thirty years later: she wanted to attain a deeper understanding
of herself and the world, without knowing where to start. Determined not to be swallowed by the dark, irrational inner world of
her mother, she clung to science, to reason. At seventeen, she met
a well-known architect, thirteen years her senior. "I was still at
school, gearing up for my final exams," she tells me. "I often spent
the lunchbreak at his place. He would make us eggs with cheese
sauce and garlic and then drop me back at school. My breath reeked
to high heaven, but I couldn't have cared less. It was as if all life's
boundaries had fallen away and the world was laid out before me.
He took me to Venice, to Rome. The world was more fun than I
could ever have imagined. And I got to be part of it all. I was seen."

Sjuwke ran her up a pale-blue wedding dress from a length of
corduroy. On the eve of her big day, my mother sighed that she
didn't really want to get married after all. Racked with doubt, she
worried that she was too young. "Life isn't about what you want,"
Sjuwke told her. And so my mother became a bride who struggled
not to look like a sulky teenager. On honeymoon in Venice, she
had her first panic attack.

The couple had a few good years together. But after a while,
he began to irritate her. "We were at our best when he was the
father and I was the daughter," she says. "We never managed the

transition to an equal relationship." Admiration soon slumped into disappointment and at twenty-four, my mother was both a university student and a young divorcée, free to look as sulky as she saw fit. Being divorced at such a tender age made her something of a novelty. A leading periodical of the day interviewed her about the phenomenon of "new-style divorce" – the "newness" presumably being that the split had been initiated by the wife and not the husband. One of the copy editors on that article was a journalist from Brabant whose sympathies lay firmly with the abandoned spouse, who he felt "had been buried under an avalanche of convoluted chatter". Although he didn't know it at the time, the journalist would go on to play his own part in this story.

Having refused alimony, my mother had to generate an income of her own, and fast. She became an assistant to Joop Goudsblom and Abram de Swaan, two charismatic sociologists who were making a name for themselves. Alongside her sociology degree, she took a sculpture course at Amsterdam's prestigious Rietveld Academy and played in a music ensemble with a penchant for light classical. She lived in a succession of draughty top-floor flats in the cramped courtyards of the Jordaan and went to bed late, usually after a night of drinking, playing chess and smoking roll-ups at a local bar. She held her own as the only woman in the male-dominated sociological circles in which she moved but it came at a price: the pressure she put on herself was considerable. Something was gnawing away at her, a feeling she countered by reading even more and working even harder.

Until one day she couldn't work at all. A cycle began in which months of intense activity were followed by inevitable collapse. Books went unread and she could no longer bring herself to see friends. She curled up under a blanket and found comfort in listening to Erik Satie on repeat, only getting up to go to the toilet and turn the record over. The notion of hours and days disappeared completely; time became a matter of side A and side B. She felt like she had "no ground beneath her feet". Even now, her sentences crumble when she talks about it. "Was afraid ... couldn't cope with life. Things that once helped fell away, lost their shine. Fear of the outside world amplified the fear on the inside, and vice versa." Turn the record over. "I knew I'd get through it eventually, but that was more something I kept telling myself, not a real conviction." From B back to A. "Looked a mess, bags under my eyes. Always on the verge of tears. Couldn't really touch the world, like there was glass between, some kind of veil." It took her weeks to scramble back to her feet. The lead-up, the tunnel, the glimmer at the end: that was the cycle.

It was her boss Abram de Swaan, a man whose ambitions bridged both sociology and psychology, who recommended she try psychoanalysis. Or did she want to repeat the same pattern her entire life, tumbling into the same pitfalls?

Psychoanalysis was the method pieced together by Sigmund Freud, an approach he believed should occupy a "middle position between medicine and philosophy". For Freud, psychoanalysis was like field research: it allowed him to test his theories while making new discoveries, which he then integrated into his theoretical corpus. And so, little by little, Freud changed our idea of fear for ever.

Exasperated by the vagueness of the term "neurasthenia", which encompassed a whole host of psychological symptoms, Freud came up with the concept of anxiety neurosis in 1894 and identified the core symptom as "anxious expectation". In doing so, he reached back, perhaps unknowingly, to two long-standing traditions: one that saw fear as a malady of the imagination and one that saw it as a response to impending harm. Freud's greatest influence on the history of fear is what became known as his "second theory of anxiety", in which fear is taken as a signal, the conscious mind's response (Freud spoke in terms of the ego) in situations where a traumatic situation is imminent and needs to be avoided. Phobias offer a highly specific example of this mechanism: people feeling fear at the sight of an ostensibly harmless object or creature, such as a spider or mouse.

Freud hypothesised that the seeds of this problem often lay in unprocessed sexual arousal, one of the many urges we feel as children which have no place in adult life. This explains why Freud, once an aspiring neuroscientist who conducted laboratory studies on the brain to find out where insanity lurked within that lobed lump of dull grey matter, had such a strong focus on early childhood. He saw gasping for air, a common side-effect of anxiety and panic, as a distant echo of our crying out at birth. A contemporary and close associate of Freud, Otto Rank, went even further. Rank maintained that anxiety was caused by the trauma of birth, a theory even Freud found speculative – by no means a recommendation. A leitmotif in Freud's thinking is the Oedipus situation: the danger in the real world is the possessive father, King Laius, who orders the death of his new-born son in response to a prophecy that the boy would one day kill his father and marry his own mother (i.e. the king's wife). As Freud saw it, the fear that this paternal threat ignited in the young Oedipus is something we all feel to a greater or lesser extent.

Before Freud, many types of fear and psychological conditions in which fear played a key role had been described in detail, but the idea that our fears originate deep within us was completely new. It seems obvious to us today, but this tends to be true of insights so revolutionary that they changed our way of thinking for ever. Yet in spite of this, the modern view of anxiety as a separate medical category, recast as a disorder in its own right, would probably have struck Freud as odd. For Freud, fear was the small change, the *Scheidemünze*, of any inner conflict.

When my mother was a schoolgirl, psychoanalysis was widely frowned upon as idle dabbling. But during her student years, it gained in prestige, coincidentally in the very sociological circles in which she found herself. Her own bosses, De Swaan and Goudsblom, took a genuine interest. It is also worth noting that the dividing line between psychiatry and psychoanalysis was also less rigid than it is today, to the point where all psychiatrists of repute at the time were also psychoanalysts. (The first DSM was published back in 1952, but it would be decades before it became a standard work.) My mother's friends were bemused by her willingness to expose herself to a regime of wild Freudian speculation and over-sexed symbolism. But she had a powerful need for a coherent narrative to account for her experience of life. And surely her bosses knew what they were talking about?

I call my mother one afternoon. Her first reaction is to assume there's something wrong, the same reaction I have whenever she calls me. I tell her about the journey I am on. About my trip to Jakarta and Bandung, my look back at the lives of Jaap Kunst and Sjuwke, her mother. But I also have a favour to ask: I would dearly like to find out more about that explanatory narrative of hers.

*

One damp Thursday evening, the moment of truth is upon us. We settle in at the Amsterdam arts society where my grandfather was a member. He died here, at his favourite table, where he liked to tuck in to the dish of the day. In front of me is the typescript of my mother's case history, errors dabbed out with Tippex. Having requested a copy of her file years before, she recently came across it during a spring clean and has agreed to go through it with me. The more sexually charged passages have been blanked out with blue marker, which gives the document the aura of an FBI memorandum. Holding a sheet up to the light, the word "orgasm" leaps out at me. I turn the pages with sweaty palms. My cup of coffee is swiftly followed by a glass of wine.

It is a curious sensation to read about the woman your mother used to be. As a child, it's easy to see yourself as the culmination of a narrative: the timelines of your parents' biographies converging in you to find their supposed high point. This narcissistic illusion is rudely undermined when you come face to face with reality: your mother could easily have lived a different life, gone on to have a completely different child or never have children at all.

Leafing through the pages that reveal my mother as seen through the eyes of the analyst charged with assessing her suitability for therapy, she appears before me as an insecure young woman. The analyst describes her as "a woman with regular features, lightly tinted glasses with metal frames, corduroy jacket, on the shabby side. Note: varnish on the nails of her left hand, but not the right." Why this is noteworthy remains unclear; the analyst's tone is as vague as it is suggestive. They clearly had no rapport. Further on, he calls her "confused, dishevelled, restless, irritable". From another session: "Today she got lost on her way here. Called me from a chip shop in completely the wrong part of town."

As for what ailed her, she had "trouble coping with life". "Always felt inadequate." She had "suicidal thoughts, to the point of obsession. Never the urge to act on them, but compelling thoughts." In addition, she struggled with "a deep-seated loneliness". She was afraid of losing control, experienced "a profound fear of having to give up her autonomy". She described her mother, Sjuwke, as "a housewife, compassionate, very warm-hearted, a gift for drawing but does nothing with it. Rather unstable." "Mother has periods of great instability: becomes very forgetful, gets confused, needs reassurance." Sjuwke's story of giving up her aspirations in order to marry had become a cautionary tale. My mother intended to do things differently.

I read on. "She is afraid of all forms of addiction, also of falling in love." Physically, she was completely worn out. The word "depressed" occurs frequently, occasionally preceded by the word "chronically". And then there was fear, which came in many guises. Abundant fear of failure. She made a "wavering, indecisive" impression. "Anxiety attacks, with muscle spasms that make all my limbs tremble." She often felt "threatened without knowing why".

Fear runs like a river through my mother's narrative. As a child, she noted in her diary that she was afraid of being "ugly, podgy, with a crooked nose, that no-one would want me". She was afraid of monsters, of demons under the bed. Afraid of being stupid, of leaving the safety of home. Other children frightened her, she hated parties. At the same time, she was highly driven: "No time to waste (aged 8 to 14)!" I read things I never even knew. Her first boyfriend drowned and her second was suicidal, as was her first lover after the divorce. I read about great aunts who killed themselves or were institutionalised for life. Despite all this, the file reassures more than it unsettles. Her symptoms are so similar to mine, it's like looking in a mirror; a mirror set at an angle, but even so. In a strange way, I have rarely felt as connected to her as I do here and now, reading about her desperate twenties. Then comes the sentence that could be read as the first spark of my life. "I do want children but haven't felt ready." *Haven't*. The tentative realisation that she might one day be ready had dawned. That hope, the benefit of the doubt, would grow steadily stronger in the years that followed until, thirteen years after lying on this analyst's couch, she would become pregnant at the age of thirty-six.

As the intake sessions progressed, the analyst's assumptions became more rigorous. "She is very insecure and vulnerable; easily anxious and out of sorts. Blushes frequently; almost appears to be daydreaming." Yet at other times, it seems she was very much on the ball. "She continues to overwhelm and rattle me." His final summing up is surprisingly aggressive. "She toys with me and uses all sorts to this end, including her insecurity [. . .] Phallic." Yep, phallic: penis-related. Sentences later, this is expanded to "phallic narcissism". Suddenly, my mother is landed with a "murderous rage towards the male", a diversion from the "murderous rage towards mother". For the record, not a single biographical detail from the file seems to back this up. "In phallic functioning," the analyst concludes, "the patient can finally reconcile herself to the fact that she was born a woman." We stare at each other in silence, then burst out laughing and order more wine.

My mother finally got the go-ahead from the intake analyst and was allowed to proceed with analysis proper. So what exactly did she learn from the twelve hundred hours she spent on the couch?

The insight that fear and hubris, the two poles between which she was constantly flung, were not each other's opposite. They belonged together. That realisation, she says, made her "feel more whole as a person". Grateful for the school of thought which had laid bare (or constructed) her personal genesis from chaos, she decided to return the favour and record the genesis of psychoanalysis in the Netherlands. It became the doctoral dissertation with which she rounded off her university years, her time of fear and hubris. It was published in 1984, two years before I was born.

In the lead-up to my birth, both my mother and my grandmother Sjuwke lived in fear. There were rational fears, about the prospect of a breech birth. Two weeks before I was born, my mother wrote in her diary: "Scared today, feel unwell. Dreading the delivery. He is still in the breech position [. . .] Why can't he just be normal?" But there were irrational fears too. In the final weeks of her pregnancy, she noted: "Fears keep rearing their heads, 'forces' getting stronger: feeling defenceless, at the mercy of others, their desires, requests, their aggression." And fears about my grandmother: "Poor Sjuw is losing her way again. Odd fears, like the needle snapping when she was making a patchwork quilt for the baby. Shaking it out, checking the fabric, nothing can put her at ease: she keeps on and on about it, till she drives you to distraction and you tell her to stop, which she can't bear, so you end up feeling guilty for lashing out at someone so kind as to make a quilt for your baby."

Then, on 20 January, 1986, a simple exclamation: "Gave birth!"

Since I came into the world, my mother has suffered fewer breakdowns. Not that my arrival cured her or anything that poetic. She continued to have her periods of fragility. When she took her to bed, I was not encouraged to go upstairs. And if I had to, it was best to tiptoe past her bedroom. I am not the healer but the runner who has taken over the baton.

# 5

## Bloodlines and Soundbites

A trail of fear runs from Indonesia to Amsterdam, through Jaap Kunst to my grandmother Sjuwke, from my grandmother to my mother, and from my mother to me. A trail I was barely aware of until I started looking. Yet my footprints fit perfectly into theirs.

A number of labels have surfaced so far: neurasthenia, melancholy, depression, phallic narcissism. Each period comes with its own repertoire of feelings, its own language in which words take on specific connotations, a weight and a texture that each patient has to find ways to accommodate. But do these different labels refer to distinct disorders? This strikes me as unlikely. My mother's psychological vulnerability was that of my grandmother, who can trace her vulnerability back to my great-grandfather Jaap. All of them instinctively obeyed the inner urge that drove them down a "path set out by inclination and disposition" and were overcome at regular intervals by the fear of not being able to cope. In short, it's the diagnoses, not the people, who change. But how should we characterise the trail that leads from Jaap to me, here, today?

The books I took to Indonesia and those forwarded from the Vallée de Misère have been reintegrated in my library of fear in Amsterdam, spilling from slightly sagging shelves to form uneven piles on the floor. Alone in my study, I am free to renew my search in the hope that it might stop me from moping over D., from reliving our scene in the kitchen. No such luck. I open my notebooks to find a string of failed letters, one unsent draft after another. Variations on a theme: I understand her reasons and hope she will find her way back to me. But, browsing further, the emphasis shifts towards passages from scientific studies on fear, notes that steer me towards the eternal question of nature versus nurture. As human beings, are we shaped primarily by our genes (nature) or by our social circumstances (nurture)? And how are these factors reflected in me?

A potted history might not go amiss at this point. In the first half of the twentieth century, it seemed like a foregone conclusion: nurture took precedence over nature. Under the influence of Freud and his kindred spirits, the environment in which a person grew up was seen as determining the course of their life. Roughly speaking, a person who had suffered no trauma and was not riven by profound inner conflicts or unresolved Oedipal tendencies (lust for mother or territorial warfare with father) would have every chance of living a well-balanced life. Freud also took a relational view of heredity, believing that shared traits and psychological characteristics among family members were a product of upbringing. Nurture, in other words.

Generally speaking, the resurgence of nature began in 1953, when James Watson, Francis Crick, Maurice Wilkins and Rosalind Franklin determined the molecular structure of DNA. Their discovery, the double helix, was published in *Nature* on 25 April, 1953. Following this Nobel-Prize-winning breakthrough, it took until the 1970s before the first serious genetic studies of psychological traits were conducted, without much success, it must be said. It wasn't until the 1980s that things really took off, as researchers began to ask which of our traits are determined by heredity.

Two research methods are best suited to answering that question: adoption studies and twin studies. The underlying rationale is clear enough. First-degree relatives – parents and children, siblings – share 50 per cent of their DNA, while adopted children share no DNA whatsoever with their adoptive parents and non-biological siblings. Parents who adopt can therefore influence the development of their non-biological children through nurture, but not through nature.

One of the first major adoption studies was initiated in the United States in the late 1970s: the Colorado Adoption Project or CAP. The results, which began to emerge in the 1980s, were nothing short of revolutionary. In practical terms, the adopted children studied turned out to resemble their biological parents far more closely than their non-biological parents, the people under whose roof and according to whose rules they had been raised. Weight, intelligence, verbal abilities, spatial understanding, memory, as well as temperament and life choices – including alcohol consumption and likelihood of divorce – turned out to be largely genetically determined. Even the time a child spent watching TV was much more consistent with the viewing habits of its biological parents than with those of its adoptive parents, though the children in the study had been less than a week old when they were given up for adoption.

The second significant step in the nature-versus-nurture debate came with the study of twins. From a genetic perspective, identical twins are especially worth studying: since they come from the same fertilised egg, their DNA is a 100 per cent match. Although it is rare for identical twins to be separated early in life, this group is of exceptional interest to scientists: what better way to find out whether behaviour can be explained genetically than by studying two genetically identical individuals who have grown up in completely different circumstances? An early example of this type of study concerns the "Jim Twins" as they were known: identical twin brothers given up for adoption a few weeks after their birth in 1940. When reunited for the first time in 1979, both brothers turned out to be six feet tall and weigh 180 pounds. Both were lousy at spelling and good at maths, and both liked carpentry and drawing. Their life paths also revealed bizarre similarities. Both had been married twice, first to a woman named Linda, then to a Betty. They were both nail biters, suffered from migraines and were heavy smokers of the same brand of cigarettes: Salem. Both men drove a light-blue Chevrolet, worked in the security industry and were father to a son. One brother had called his boy James Alan, the other had opted for James Allan.

Another study that produced compelling results was the Twins Early Development Study or TEDS, a wide-ranging British twins study from the 1990s that took in more than sixteen thousand families. It found that identical twins who grew up separately were almost as similar as identical twins who grew up together. Here too, nature proved far more powerful than nurture. The study also established that identical twins were much more alike than non-identical twins; that may sound blindingly obvious but it would not apply unless genetic differences were a factor of significance. These similarities went much deeper than outward appearance: reading ability, verbal skills, general learning and spatial understanding were all found to be largely genetically determined.

As the number of adoption and twins studies grew in the 1990s, so did the scientific conviction that a person's genes have a major influence on their character, temperament and mental stability. In the scientific literature, lack of mental stability is linked with neuroticism, a term so closely associated with anxious tendencies that many scientists use "neuroticism" and "anxiety" interchangeably. Neuroticism is a personality trait that leaves a person more open to anxiety, more sensitive to stress and more prone to powerful negative emotions such as nervousness, sadness and anger. The higher your score on the neuroticism scale, the more susceptible you are to anxiety disorders, burnout and depression. Jaap Kunst, my highly strung great-grandfather springs to mind immediately.

Turning the spotlight on fear, it was not until the 1980s that this approach was specifically applied to people with excessive anxiety, with interesting results. Geneticist Sven Torgersen carried out a study of all Norwegian twins who had been diagnosed with an anxiety disorder. According to his findings, published in 1983, the risk of both twins developing an anxiety disorder was three times higher in identical twins than in non-identical or dizygotic twins: 45 compared to 15 per cent. Most meta-analyses – large-scale research that surveys the results of a range of scientific studies – have shown that the risk of developing either an anxiety disorder or depression is four to six times greater for someone with a first-degree relative who suffers from one of these conditions. The estimated heritability of both is between 30 and 50 per cent. To be clear, this is not an unambiguous victory for the nature camp: these findings still put 50 to 70 per cent of the risk of a disorder beyond the realm of genetics.

What is the genetic difference between an anxiety disorder and depression? It's an intriguing question that I have repeatedly put to doctors and other experts through the years. No wonder I had trouble getting a straight answer: there appears to be no incontrovertible distinction. The genes that affect one disorder also affect the other. In 1987, an influential study of 3,800 sets of Australian twins led to the important insight that, while the likelihood of developing a mental disorder – the distress factor – is largely genetically determined, the form the disorder takes depends on chance environmental factors. (Previously, scientists thought the opposite: that your chance of developing a mental illness was determined by your environment, while the form it took was genetically determined.) In general, you can say that experiences of loss and grief are more likely to push you towards depression, while encountering severe danger is more likely to push you towards an anxiety disorder.

It is important to realise that no one specific gene is responsible for a particular mental disorder, a belief that geneticist and psychologist Robert Plomin has dubbed the OGOD misconception (one gene, one disorder). There is no such thing as a "depression gene". Mental disorders do not arise from a few abnormal snippets of DNA, but from tens of thousands of normal snippets of DNA which can combine in ways that adversely affect our mental health. To confuse matters further, those same "adverse" genetic combinations may even work to our benefit, enhancing certain talents or positive qualities. Being prone to anxiety, for instance, might make someone more sensitive and caring. Having what might be termed a mental abnormality therefore amounts to no more than an extreme result of a normal distribution of tens of thousands of DNA snippets that, in a given constellation, can negatively impact our mental condition. Stated more simply, everyone has a wealth of potentially detrimental genetic material; the end result is a matter of degree, not one thing or another.

All things considered, we can conclude that nature has a significant role to play in the fears that are handed down to us. In the words of Jaap Kunst, our inclinations and disposition determine the path.

*

Time to get personal again. How do these natural laws play out in my family history? I fish out the notebook that contains my family tree, the roots and branches that link Jaap, Sjuwke, my mother and me.

Jaap Kunst died many years before scientists coined the term "distress factor" but its applicability to his life story is evident. Of Jaap's three children – Sjuwke, Egbert and Japie – it was Sjuwke who was particularly prone to depression. Only two of Sjuwke's four children – my mother and my uncle – have experienced breakdowns. My mother gave birth to two sons, me and my younger brother Thomas. Neither of us are exactly what you would call the life and soul of the party, but it is only in me that the distress factor has led to regular bouts of depression and heightened anxiety. Viewed statistically, my family tree provides an almost perfect illustration of the 50 per cent rate of heritability. (I also have two half-sisters on my father's side, but since we share less genetic material and did not grow up together, I have left them out of this overview.) Of course, the paternal bloodline is also part of this story but, in my case, this is harder to pin down in relation to depression and anxiety. My father's parents were sombre people but it is difficult to say whether their demeanour was hereditary or the logical consequence of trauma: they were scarred by the loss of their daughter, killed in a road accident as a young girl. Nor do I see their chronically muted emotional life reflected in the pattern I see in myself and my mother's side of the family: the highs of a zest for life bordering on hubris giving way to deep troughs of despair.

Although my brother and I have the same parents and have had roughly the same upbringing, he is far less prone to anxiety than I am. That said, he is cautious by nature and no stranger to stress and the fear of screwing things up. On the whole then, our family's heritability rate for elevated anxiety sensitivity hovers around the 50 per cent mark. I find this genetic determinism oddly reassuring: it's as if I have simply followed the dictates of my genes, and there's a sense in which I am not to blame for my fears.

Genetics does not tell the whole story, of course, and it is mainly up to psychological research to reveal the part played by nurture. Children who grow up in the same family can lead widely differing lives. They go through different experiences, make their own friends and are taught by different teachers. Meanwhile, their own individual genetic make-up and sensibilities mean they gravitate towards different interests. These environmental variables go on to weave an additional layer of psychological difference. Negative, angry or impatient parental reactions increase a child's risk of depression later in life. If a parent is more negative towards one child than another, that child is more likely to suffer from both anxiety and depression. My brother and I have different temperaments. He is calmer and more even-tempered, more like our father. I have always been more emotional and volatile, and Dad didn't know how to respond to my outbursts. He came down harder on me than he did on my brother, a response prompted by my behaviour, which in turn was a result of my temperament. Parental inconsistencies like these nearly always feed into the family dynamic. A mother is often overprotective of an anxious child, and this can lead the father to compensate subconsciously by being stricter. This can create a completely different situation for one sibling as opposed to the other. No two families are the same and within the same family, each member has a different experience.

To further complicate the nature-versus-nurture issue, the two are intertwined and exert a constant influence on each other. Your genetic make-up influences your environment and how you experience it, but the opposite is also true. Your environment influences your genes.

The relatively new, more holistic field of research that studies this interaction is called "epigenetics", "epi" meaning "at" or "on". Epigenetics focuses on the ways in which gene expression is fine-tuned by factors that can change throughout your lifetime. In the course of your life, the expression of your genes – how they manifest themselves in your appearance or behaviour – can alter. Molecules can even be added to your DNA. In studies, rats that were frequently licked and stroked by their mothers gave the same attention to their own babies, because certain chemical groups had attached themselves to genes in the hippocampus, allowing them to instinctively recall that behaviour. Mice whose cages contained toys when they were young gave birth to offspring with more highly developed cognitive functions.

Similar processes have been observed in us humans. There are notable examples of how circumstances affect our genes, none of which have yet been explained by scientists. An extensive Swedish study found that the grandsons of men who had been malnourished during pre-adolescence were less likely to die of cardiovascular disease. A study of the male children of soldiers who had been captured and tortured in the American Civil War found that they were 10 per cent more likely to die in any given year on reaching middle age. Another American study concluded that Dutch people whose foetal development had taken place during severe food shortages towards the end of the Second World War showed a certain chemical reaction, an epigenetic signature, that made them relatively overweight later in life.

The epigenetic principle works something like this: the neurons in your brain respond to what you experience, and make proteins and enzymes which in turn attach to your genes. So even in the case of two people with an identical genetic make-up, the disparate events and experiences of their separate lives would cause their DNA to behave differently: for example, if one were exposed to greater danger or more unsafe situations growing up, a logical epigenetic response would be a rise in stress hormones because a child in those circumstances would benefit from an optimal fear system. Although the exact nature of a child's upbringing may not have a huge influence on the extent to which they develop anxiety, childhood is still key in that scientists see it as the time in our lives when most epigenetic changes occur.

Childhood. The word stays with me as I gather my things and head downstairs, having completed about a quarter of my journey. It has taught me that the division of human experience into environmental factors and a genetic component is largely artificial, not least because nature and nurture are so variously and intimately intertwined. After ploughing my way through dozens of studies, I can't help but conclude that it's a unique blend of the two that makes people more or less anxious.

In the age-old "nature versus nurture" debate it's the word "versus" that trips us up. Every scientist knows that nature and nurture are not opposing forces; they react to each other and interact in all kinds of complex ways. Unfortunately, the metaphors that make the covers of scientific bestsellers often tend towards the simplistic. Richard Dawkins and *The Selfish Gene*. Dick Swaab's insistence that *We Are Our Brains*. Dive into the books themselves and you soon see the mismatch between the conclusions their authors reach and the promotional soundbites formulated to grab the attention of the media. The depth of the actual scientific knowledge on display is one thing, but the simplifications bandied about in the ensuing public debate are something else again. However conscientious these writers are, however nuanced their discourse, once their book has topped the bestseller list, it's the soundbites the public remembers.

But my fears cannot be captured in soundbites, encapsulated by geneticists, tabulated by statisticians or summed up in scientific bestsellers. By definition, stories about fear are personal and particular; they always come down to people, to individuals who relate to their fears in an intimate way. I am no exception. Amsterdam begins to blur around the edges; a bank of mist settles over the canals as I unlock my bike. The trouble is, no story of fear is unambiguous, mine included. There are twists and turns, back alleys leading to other areas of inquiry, not to mention a cast of unlikely characters, some of whom I have known for decades.

# 6

## The Bat's Dark Shadow

"If I have a son, I will make him grow his hair long. From the age of one, he will go to a crèche. It is important that he forms attachments to as many people as possible. I will not stand for any jealousy or hostility between him and his sister because there will be no reason for it. The house will be littered with comics. A list of alternative support agencies will be stuck to the inside of his school bag; he will never have to call them. He certainly won't have to pursue a career. Studying will be by no means a must. As long as he finds a job he likes, one that will earn him a half-decent living. So that he can make something of his life. More than I have."

Spread out before me on the desk of my boyhood bedroom and smelling faintly of cigarette smoke is a yellowed copy of *Aloha*, a magazine that graced newsstands from 1969 to 1974. This editorial from the final issue entitled "If I Have a Son" was written by one of *Aloha*'s regular contributors. His Monday morning deadline meant that he always wrote his pieces on Sunday night, banging away on a mid-sized Olympia typewriter in his cramped study. Sometimes he worked so late that he was on hand to whip up a breakfast of instant porridge for his daughters. Those daughters are my half-sisters. That editor is my father. And the son he said he wanted in 1974 turned out to be me, in 1986. Perhaps this column contains the first traces of my life, the first of him as my father in any case. I sit down at the desk, gaze up at my old football shirts, competing for wall space with posters of action heroes. School textbooks still line the shelves. My father foresaw one thing perfectly in 1974: there are comics everywhere.

It's not hard to access feelings from my childhood, positive or negative, nebulous or crystal clear. The negatives are not fraught with danger – the risk of choking on a wine gum was about as perilous as things got – but steeped in uncertainty and confusion. At times, the world I was part of seemed incomprehensible to me. What were its laws, its rules, its codes? I often failed to grasp the reasoning behind what I saw and heard, a state of ignorance that left me feeling threatened. My experience of the world was characterised by an inability to impose order. The shapes in my bedroom shifted after dark. Shadows became ghosts. A pencil case twisted into an antler, a shirt thrown in the corner burst into a sea of flames. I would be afraid that my bedroom door no longer opened onto the hallway, that my room had been cut adrift and was floating free across the city. (Rationale: unclear.) I developed a sudden fear of sockets, convinced that they could swallow body parts. (Rationale: my uncle had stuck his thumb in an unearthed socket as a child and only had a stump to show for it.) I was afraid brushing my teeth would make me foam at the mouth. (Rationale: a TV villain foaming at the mouth after swallowing a cyanide pill and my father shaking his head and saying "It's only toothpaste".) Even at home, I imagined that I was vulnerable and exposed, though there was no place I felt safer. So much so that home-sickness became an issue; it was only as a teenager that – with the trepidation of someone dipping their toes in a water hole – I would occasionally sleep over at a friend's house. In a fit of pique, I might resolve to run away from home but I was never gone long.

My best friend at primary school was Jara. Too ham-fisted to tie my own shoelaces, I would shuffle over to her desk at least twice a day. As soon as she saw me coming, she would get up from her chair. This little ritual came to define my first idea of a true friend: someone who will tie your laces without having to be asked. Later, it was Jara I called when the school board threatened to expel me. I had teamed up with a pal to write a dictionary of dirty words, a puerile mix of words we had heard ("muff diver"), words we stuck together ("mordorfucker") and ones we made up ("freumpette", which meant something like "numbskull"). For days my fate hung in the balance, or so it seemed. I even stayed over at Jara's to avoid having to face my parents. Jara's dad, who had once promised me a million guilders if I managed to fill a jam jar with toe cheese, told funny, freewheeling bedtime stories. I fell asleep with his felt hat pulled down over my ears. It transpired that the school board only wanted to shake me up and had never intended to turf me out. Could I have figured that out for myself? Possibly, but fear had crippled my judgement. Even after it had all blown over, the sense of foreboding proved difficult to shrug off. I returned to school feeling like I could be sent packing at any moment and I found myself calling Jara more and more. She never called me. Once she admitted it was because she was scared that my father would answer the phone.

My father. Out of everything and everyone, I understood him least of all. No matter how hard I tried, the motives that underpinned his actions, the factors that influenced his behaviour remained a complete mystery. One thing I knew: he wasn't anxious like me. He seemed to have armoured himself against such disruptive emotions, at least that is my best guess looking back after all these years. Instead, he appeared to operate in a twilight state, impervious to fear but untouched by intense happiness. My mother, whose family history of anxiety was a big influence on me, was never a puzzle, like my father. If she was overworked, she said so; if she was happy, there was no mistaking it. She was home all day but determined less of the daily routine because she was hard at work upstairs. The living room – and the TV – were downstairs, next to my father's study.

Unpredictable is the word that sums up my boyhood impression of my father. He could be thoughtful and generous, surprising me with tickets for an Ajax game or combing the street markets on Queen's Day for Batman action figures. He would record my favourite programmes on VHS, including the 1960s *Batman* series, its tame campery given a new lease of life by a kids' channel in the early 1990s. Just before dinner – which usually consisted of pasta caked in whitish sauce or cordon bleus fried to a crisp by my mother – he would plonk himself down on the couch and we would tune in for another exciting episode, my head resting on his paunch. Or the "dad pad", as we called it.

Yet that warmth was not a constant. As a rule, he wasn't big on physical contact and would even recoil slightly if we touched him. He was often absent. When I left for school in the morning, he was asleep, having worked deep into the night. In the evenings, after *Batman* and dinner, he would usually retire to his study, his presence reduced to the rattling of his typewriter. (Work was paramount, he explained to me recently. In his eyes, it was a father's role to *be* somebody, out there in the real world. To make sure he would never be a source of shame to his children.) Through the stained-glass of the sliding doors, brown from cigarette smoke, the crackle of his portable TV could be heard, giving way to the heartfelt throb of blues music as the evening wore on. What went on in there always felt more important than anything that might occur in the living room or the kitchen. Sitting on the couch, I always wanted him to come out and sit with me. It never occurred to me to get off the couch and knock on his door. Perhaps we were waiting for each other.

So I stayed put in a living room that was steadily filling with cigarette smoke. My dodgy lungs meant that asthma attacks were a regular occurrence but if I opened a window, my father would come storming out of his study. It's like bloody Siberia in here. What was I trying to do? Drive him out of his own house? I choked on my own words, struggled to understand why he was so angry. That lack of understanding regularly exploded into tantrums, which I sometimes took out on my opponents on the football pitch. "Daan is a very intense child," my mother, then a sociology professor, said in a 1997 interview. "In everything – anger, sorrow, but also joyful anticipation. It's something we share. I was an eager child, threw myself into every pursuit. That kinship can move me, his sensitivity, that same intensity. The sense that all that you feel is too much for this life." If my father thought I was being too intense, he would cool me off by holding my head under the cold tap, his fingers and thumbs pressed to my temples. Far from cooling me off, this had me thrashing around like a madman, convinced that I couldn't breathe. (When I ask him, he tells me this happened once. As I recall, it happened more often. It's impossible to say who is right.)

One of his most vivid memories of me as a boy is in the passenger seat of the car, trembling before every football match. "We would drive out to Kudelstaart and you'd be quivering with nerves. And I had no idea why you were so tense, what you were so scared of. Scared to lose? To not play well? Afraid no-one would pass you the ball?" It was a variation on the second option: fear of disappointing my teammates. And perhaps him too.

I mentioned earlier that the specifics of parenting have little influence on whether a child becomes excessively anxious later in life. What *is* crucial, is being surrounded by a consistently warm and loving environment at an early age. This may sound obvious, but a century ago it was nothing of the sort.

In the first decades of the twentieth century, the medical consensus was that parents should refrain from touching their children too often. John Watson, head of the American Psychological Association, propagated this idea and saw it confirmed by the studies he carried out in hospitals. Watson concluded that children who were held more frequently by the nursing staff were more at risk of death than those who were not touched. Today, this would be put down to the transfer of bacteria, something that was not common knowledge at the time. "Mother love is a dangerous instrument," was the view he expressed in 1928. And he was not alone. At the time, the US government distributed pamphlets warning against the dangers of holding your child. "Never hug and kiss them, never let them sit in your lap," Watson warned, predicting a troubled life ahead for the child who was kissed too often. "Too often" meant more than once a year.

It was the 1950s before Watson's ideas were completely refuted, thanks to the attachment theory formulated by British psychiatrist John Bowlby. After studying the work of the first ethologists (animal behaviour scientists) in the preceding decades, it occurred to Bowlby that humans and animals might not differ as much as was widely assumed: after all, infant primates exhibited roughly the same attachment behaviour as human babies. He reasoned that healthy attachment at an early age served an important evolutionary purpose, improving a young ape's chances of survival as it learned to control its impulses and identify danger more accurately. It is a view that also lends a Darwinian dimension to separation anxiety: the ape that forms the closest attachment to its mother has the best chance of survival. Bowlby carried his ideas over into a long-term study of juvenile delinquents, many of whom had bonded poorly or not at all with their parents (especially their mothers). As a result, they had acquired no "internal working model" of parental love, no internalised sense of appreciation and security. They had been left without a secure foundation from which to explore life.

Over the course of his long career, Bowlby, aided by psychologist Mary Ainsworth, formulated three attachment types. Secure attachment – a successful, warm bond with parents – statistically led to few subsequent feelings of anxiety and a healthy relationship with intimacy. Ambivalent attachment – an erratic bond with the parents, often manifested in dependent behaviour by the child – was a predictor of high levels of anxiety in adult life. Avoidant attachment – a distant bond with parents, often resulting in deviant and unpredictable behaviour – was an indicator of an aversion to intimacy in adult life. Although Bowlby's ideas came in for ongoing criticism from psychoanalytic quarters, where comparing humans to animals was taboo, scientific studies have repeatedly vindicated the principles underlying his ideas. (Those same ideas have also had unfortunate side effects, with mothers feeling pressured or guilty if they feel they are not offering their child a healthy degree of attachment.)

Modern neurological research has also lent support to attachment theory in interesting ways. Jaak Panksepp, a revolutionary Estonian-American neurobiologist, devoted years of his career to researching the neurological basis for our emotions. He concluded, after painstaking studies which involved sliding electrodes millimetre by millimetre across the skulls of his subjects, that the human brain has seven systems, all operating and interacting simultaneously. Four of those systems are positive. The *seeking* system prompts foraging behaviour and stimulates our desire to go out into the wide world. The *lust* system leads to sexual desire. The *care* system encourages us look after each other. And then there is the *play* system, which encourages us to fool around and have fun. The three negative systems he identified were *fear*, *panic/grief* and *rage*. At this point, I should make a slight amendment to something I said earlier: while our fear system resembles that of the rat, there are also differences. The system that drives our biological response to danger, our fight-or-flight response, is the same. But unlike the rat, we also have a panic system, in which attachment plays a major role. Roughly speaking, if you feel unsafe in your attachment and never really learn to put your trust in others, you will be more inclined towards panic.

Watching *Batman* with my dad is the safest I have ever felt. The caped crusader came in the shape of Adam West, a wooden actor who had pulled on a pair of shiny blue swimming trunks over a light-grey body suit. Every blow he dealt was shielded from my impressionable young eyes by an explosion of brightly coloured graphics: Kaboom! Pow! Bang! Dad taped every episode so I could watch them on repeat, something I did daily. And, having absorbed each one, frame by frame, if there was anything I didn't understand, I simply wrote to the TV. One letter, from 1991, concerned the unfathomable (and therefore unsettling) transition when Bruce Wayne and Dick Grayson leap onto two fire poles on the first floor of Wayne Manor and slide into the Batcave in the very next shot as Batman and Robin:

> Dear Telekids,
> Batman starts off normal, but when he comes off the pole he has his suit on. How does that work? Where does he get changed? My name is Daan. I watch every-every-every day. Dear Batman, dear Robin, I can say "yes" and "no" and "let's go" too. Dear Telekids. Dear commissioner.

When my friends asked me what I wanted to be when I grew up, I always answered "Batman".

A friend of my mother's who was a dab hand at sewing transformed a length of cotton into a bat cape and stapled two pieces of felt together for a mask. I liked the way the staples jagged my ears. Black sweatpants and a black jumper with the Batman logo completed my get-up. I insisted on going to school dressed like this, even in the summer, much to my mother's despair: not the coolest of outfits in any sense. At dinner time, I would astound one and all by appearing out of nowhere, bat wings spread wide. This actually meant popping out from behind the curtains, where I had been gently braising in the smells of Mum's cooking for at least half an hour, my feet presumably giving my top-secret location away to anyone who glanced in my general direction.

I often fantasised about becoming Batman. For me, he was the only superhero who invited that possibility. Perseverance, imagination and money were what set him apart, three things anyone could attain if they tried hard enough. Looking back on his years as a bat, Adam West mused that everyone wanted to be Batman: the man whose wife is stolen from him; the parent whose child is bullied. Everyone who thinks, "If only I were that little bit stronger, that little bit braver". As he saw it, we all have something of the avenger, the vigilante in us.

I no longer remember whether I recognised the link between Batman and fear, or how much I understood about own my fears back then. Very little, I would imagine. Yet it's hard for me to dismiss the appeal as pure coincidence: out of all the superheroes, I identified obsessively with the only one whose *raison d'être* is fear.

The relationship between fear and daring, between passivity and aggression, was a prime concern for nineteenth- and twentieth-century philosophers, at a time when fear had yet to be consigned to the realm of illness. They considered these issues without being able to reference Batman, the perfect illustration of what they wanted to say. Today, a visitor in my own boyhood bedroom, I pick up a battered comic about Batman's early years and begin to read. As with Thomas Aquinas, Avicenna and Robert Burton, Batman's story of fear starts with a plank.

*

One day, young Bruce Wayne is playing in the garden at Wayne Manor. A plank over an old well gives way beneath him and he tumbles into a cave. Silence, darkness. And then, an explosion: piercing shrieks, the frantic rush of beating wings. It is not long before Bruce's father, Thomas, finds him and hoists him back up to the surface. "Why do we fall?" the father asks and then answers for his son: "So we can learn to pick ourselves up."

But when Thomas Wayne hits the ground, he does not get back up. A few months after plunging into the well, young Bruce accompanies his parents to the opera. The sight of black-clad dancers spinning and tumbling in the sinister decor catapults him back to the shrieking torrent of bats in the cave. Thomas reads the panic in his impressionable son's eyes and decides it's time to go. They leave the theatre through a side exit that opens onto Park Row, an alley of rusted fire escapes, torn garbage bags and iron grates hissing steam. A shadowy figure approaches, pulls out a gun and demands Thomas's wallet and his wife Martha's jewellery. "That's fine," Thomas says. "Take it easy. Here you go." But as he hands over his wallet, it falls to the ground. The gunman twitches and clasps his weapon with both hands. Thomas steps sideways to shield his wife and, panicked, the man pulls the trigger, hitting Thomas square in the chest. Martha screams. Another shot rings out and her screaming stops. The man snatches at Martha's necklace but the string snaps and, as pearls skitter across the wet cobbles, he disappears into the shadows again. Bruce kneels at his father's side. Glassy-eyed, Thomas looks up at his son and whispers one final word of advice: "Bruce . . . Don't be afraid."

The orphaned son spends years pondering his father's final words. As a student, Bruce reads the work of philosopher Søren Kierkegaard, who insists that every human being experiences "an unrest, an inner strife, a disharmony, an anxiety about an unknown something [. . .] an anxiety about some possibility in existence or an anxiety about himself". Fear as the foreshadowing of freedom, of possibilities, of choices. For Kierkegaard, fear entailed acknowledging your potential and offered you the chance to become yourself. This idea is akin to what psychoanalyst Otto Rank called "fear of life": the fear of the profound changes you initiate as you develop. Rank juxtaposed fear of life with fear of death, or rather fear of nothingness. As he saw it, each person carries these two fears within them, and mental health comes down to finding a balance and accepting them both.

"Anxiety may be compared with dizziness," Kierkegaard wrote. Fear is what you experience when you look down into an abyss, a dizzying surge of disorientation that can feel almost euphoric. The abyss is terrifying but also holds an appeal: it draws you closer, you want to look. Like a child terrified by horror stories who – perhaps for that very reason – wants to hear more. The abyss became a favoured metaphor for Kierkegaard; it symbolised the distance between who we are (our reality on this side of the abyss) and who we can be (our potential, on the far side). What you need to do, Kierkegaard argues, what every human being needs to do to throw off their chains and become completely themselves, is to jump. Kierkegaard's complex work on fear is tricky to summarise but, as I see it, that leap need not be heroic or active. It may simply involve letting go of the existing certainties in your life. At that time, Bruce had yet to read Sartre, who associated fear of the abyss less with the attempt to leap across and more with the idea that you could allow yourself to fall in.

As a student, Bruce neither jumps nor falls. Every year, he returns to the alley where his parents were gunned down and leaves two red roses, one for each bullet fired. Then comes the night where he stows away on a cargo ship and disappears. The crew allow him to do menial work in exchange for his keep, but if any of them bait or insult him, Bruce flies at them. In these fits of rage, he discovers, his fears disappear for a while. When the ship docks on foreign shores, Bruce begins a nomadic existence. If there is no work to be had, he steals to survive. A night spent in jail invariably ends in a brawl.

Years pass before he returns home, by which time the city is in the grip of organised crime. Law enforcement and the judiciary are on the criminal payroll and the few who have not bowed to corruption are afraid to speak out. One night, Bruce heads for the East End, collar up, hat pulled low. A dangerous place of neon-lit streets, sex clubs, hard liquor, drunks hunched in filthy alleyways, girls smoking on corners. A sweet-spoken voice says, "Want me to show you a good time, Mister?" A girl with stud earrings, red lipstick, hands on her hips. Bruce asks her how old she is.

"As young as you want me to be."

A wiry man in a grey suit appears out of nowhere and grabs

her, his fierce eyes fixed on Bruce from under the brim of a film-noir Homburg. "You stink of cop," he sneers. Onlookers crowd round. The man pulls a stiletto. No stranger to unarmed combat, Bruce dodges the blade and floors his attacker with a well-aimed kick and a knee to the groin. But Bruce has forgotten the girl, who retrieves the stiletto from the gutter and drives it into his thigh.

Kicking and punching his way through the assembled gawkers, Bruce makes it back to Wayne Manor, a place that still feels very much like his parents' home, not his. Bloodied and bruised, he collapses onto a chair in the study, opposite a bust of Thomas. Confronted with his dead father's stony stare, a new wave of fear grips him.

This is when I imagine Bruce coming face to face with the core of anxiety as defined by Martin Heidegger (whose work is even trickier to summarise than Kierkegaard's): the awareness of the impossibility inherent in every life. The impossibility of living for ever, of avoiding death. Our end is fixed. In Heidegger's view, we all need to take that leap, to engage with the terrifying realisation of insignificance, to experience the reality that your life too will end in nothingness. Only by confronting that nothingness, that fear, can you shoulder the burden that comes with it: that you and you alone determine how your life will proceed. Only by taking that responsibility can you become an *authentic individual*, a fully formed *actual person*. To sidestep this confrontation is to remain a nameless part of the inglorious, soulless, mediocre masses.

Bruce can't stop thinking about his parents. About the hundreds of lives they might have led, lives swallowed by that single outcome: nothingness, two bodies rotting in the cold, hard earth. Only then does he see the trail of blood he has left across the floor. Perhaps he too will die in the knowledge that he never found his path. Still, better off dead than spending another hour in the quiet despair that has been his companion since that night in the alley, eighteen years before. Ever since, there has been nothing to hold the pieces of his life together. If only there were a symbol, something to believe in.

Why hadn't those East End lowlifes been afraid of him? "God . . ." he mumbles, dizzy from losing so much blood. "Fear . . . have to find a way to scare them . . ." At that moment a bat bursts through the window, vampire wings reflected from all angles in the shards of glass flying through the air. The same creature that had terrified him in the cave beneath the well, the same fear that had forced him and his parents out of the opera house and into the alley that night.

The bat lands on the stone effigy of his father's face.

"Yes, Father," Bruce says, as if giving in to something. "I must be able to strike terror into their hearts. I shall become a bat."

The transformation takes place in the dark, in the dank vaults beneath Wayne Manor. Down among those caves teeming with bats, he establishes his base of operations. He hatches plans, designs a suit and installs powerful computers to aid him in his detective work. Whenever his sense of purpose deserts him, he heads deeper into the caves, spreads his arms and stands in a maelstrom of wings.

By day he is Bruce Wayne, a devil-may-care rich man's son whose life revolves around fast cars and beautiful women; by night he is Batman, the dark knight who avenges all manner of crime with violent retribution. Wayne and Batman exchange masks with ever increasing frequency, for years on end. He grows old in that suit. "Maybe I didn't become Batman to fight crime," he says one night in despair. "Maybe it was to fight that fear."

"And instead, you became the fear," his faithful retainer Alfred observes.

"If that's true, then Batman is my enemy," Bruce replies. "Can I give up? Can I leave the shadows? And if I do, who am I?"

\*

I put the comic away. I grew up with Batman, and he grew up with me. As he matured, I made frantic attempts to do the same. That was no mean feat. Looking back at my school days, I see two boys relating to their fear in opposing ways.

Boy No. 1 was plagued by anxiety attacks for the first three years of high school: trembling, teary-eyed, short of breath. There were even blackouts. Exams sent me into a tailspin. I became notorious. When I bumped into a former teacher a few years ago, he recalled invigilating a class test, having been warned beforehand that one of the boys would probably freak out. If that happened, he was to reassure him as best he could and offer him the chance to repeat the test at a later date. That boy was me. Many a classmate dismissed my behaviour as a ploy to obtain preferential treatment, but the prospect of having to endure this misery all over again was usually enough to coax me back to my desk. "And sure enough . . .!" the teacher grinned that sunny afternoon, almost twenty years after the fact.

Those surges of panic seethed with worries and pitch-black scenarios, one dark thought triggering the next. On and on they ran, every minor setback a foreshadowing of the end. And when a surge subsided, there was the fear that it would be back to haunt me before long. *It*. This thing. The monster. The old enemy. Was I so very different from my classmates? I wondered. Was I strange, or even insane? That question opened the door to a new, underlying fear: of one day losing the battle, of being driven mad by my fears, unable to claw my way back to solid ground. I had no idea what that fateful moment would look like. A silent-movie scene involving a van and men flapping about in long white coats? Or a halting conversation between two lovers, in the kitchen of a home they once shared?

At high school, fear began to talk to me, to feed me the same line it still whispers on a daily basis: you're not going to make it. Exactly what "making it" or "not making it" means is something I have yet to figure out. The manifestation of the fear, the exact phrasing of its whispered message is constantly changing. At school, "not making it" meant having to repeat a year if I failed my exams (a quirk of the Dutch school system). The few friends you have will move on and you will remain behind to face your fears alone. I had friends, decent lads with dependable names like Sam, John and Danny, friends who reassured me, told me not to be afraid. The day before an exam, I could talk to one or two of them for hours on the phone, hang up and then call back fifteen minutes later, as if the previous conversation had never taken place. I clung to them. There was a compulsive, almost ritualistic aspect to our friendship. Always doing the same things at the same times: two hours of football on Saturday afternoon, cycling to school together. I have no idea if they knew how important they were to me. Teachers didn't know how to handle this frightened, volatile kid. I had sessions with the school psychologist, with a specialist in fear of failure, with mentors who helped me plan my studies. Nothing seemed to make a difference. I began to think I was at the wrong school. I felt too stupid, too scared, couldn't bear being so reliant on others. The school board ignored my pleas for a transfer.

Boy No. 2 arrived on the scene around my fifteenth birthday. Something in me changed. Perhaps it was the transition from lower to upper school and the prospect of a clean slate, surrounded by classmates who had never seen me throw up, cave in under pressure or burst into tears. Who had never looked on in amazement as I sprinted out of the classroom for no apparent reason. My new classmates were not model students, and this freed me from a stifling sense of competition. Better still, they were always up for a spot of mischief. At breaktime, we would smoke a joint in the park or play drinking games. I began turning up late for class, sometimes stoned and/or drunk. Often, I didn't bother turning up at all. Shoplifting became a routine after-school pastime. To this day, I feel a pang of shame looking back on those pilfered granola bars, but it wasn't about the spoils or the bragging rights. I wanted to prove to myself that I wasn't a hostage to fear, some-thing I achieved by doing things I had no real desire to do, like stealing. At the time I had never heard of counterphobic behaviour: the urge to seek out what you fear, in my case fear itself. The unfiltered anxiety of the first three years of high school made way for its opposite: putting up a stupid, unruly and destructive front. With hindsight, it's hard not to see this radical transformation as an attempt to wipe out the boy I had been for the previous three years. The kid choked by fear desperately wanting to be the kid everyone else is afraid of.

On leaving school, I fled to Italy. (Not as a cargo-ship stowaway unfortunately, nor did I return to a cave full of bats.) Strolling through my college town or looking out over the green valley dotted with turrets, white walls and red-tiled roofs, I would sometimes start to gasp for breath. If the anxiety grew overwhelming, I pressed the blade of a small knife into the flesh of my arms and legs. This had the effect of blocking fears and doubts by confronting me with a sensation of a completely different order, a sharpness that was perfectly concrete and clear, a physical pain that left no room for thoughts or machinations. After a year in Italy, I fled back home, hoping everything would be different, that I was different.

As a student in Amsterdam, I didn't fare much better. If I hit a particularly bad patch, I would go to see the father of my old friend Jara, a psychiatrist. The first time I sat trembling in his office, I asked him if he had managed to set that million guilders aside. He shot me a puzzled look. "For my toe cheese," I explained. A vague glimmer of recognition and a shake of the head. No reward money for me. "Divorce is an expensive hobby," he confided. On a wing and a prayer, pretty much, he wrote me a series of prescriptions. These remedies worked, tempering my anxiety but also putting a damper on my inner life as a whole.

Sometimes I had recourse to parental support. Whenever I knocked on my father's door, he would take me on a drive to a nearby village: Ouderkerk aan de Amstel or Monnickendam. I remember fog, rain, chomping salted herring in a village square. He made time for me. A man who is good in a crisis. At times,

I think a crisis is the only situation he completely trusts, that lets him know exactly what is required of him.

*

In short, my teens and my student years were dominated by desperate, fumbling attempts to respond to anxiety. In the end, caving in to pressure or railing against my fears was the best I could do. At the time I was oblivious to the inextricable link between fear and aggression. Psychiatrist Carl Jung argued that there are two sides to every person: the side we present to others and the side we keep hidden, whether we realise it or not; the fearful, violent, jealous aspects of our character we would rather not acknowledge. Jung uses the image of the shadow to talk about this dark, unknown side. "Everyone carries a shadow," Jung writes, "and the less embodied in the individual's conscious life, the blacker and denser it is."

Much like the gods of ancient Greece, superheroes offer us an extreme magnification of ourselves. They battle many of the same problems we face, even if their superpowers give them access to other solutions. By splitting himself into two personalities, the billionaire playboy and the violent avenger, Bruce Wayne gave his dark side plenty of room to grow. By naming his shadow while banishing it from his everyday life, he allowed it to grow darker, denser and more aggressive. In this too, Bruce is not alone: none of us is a stranger to aggression. And many of us do not have the luxury of relating to fear as an abstract, philosophical concept, let alone the luxury of a fictional existence. For some, aggression is the only response to fear they can muster, a matter of visceral necessity. The way of the bat, where the rule of law and common decency crumbles in the face of other forces, is unfathomably dark. And where I have taken a few hapless steps, others walk on until they become hopelessly lost.

*

Biologists distinguish between two types of aggression: predatory aggression and anxiety aggression. Predatory aggression is the killer instinct that kicks in when a hunter sees its prey, or the sadism that stirs in a psychopath on encountering a defenceless being. Anxiety aggression is more ambiguous and interesting: it is the furious reaction many people exhibit when they feel threatened, in the hope that anger will deter their aggressor. This mechanism can be explained by biochemistry. An adrenaline rush drowns out the stress hormone we call cortisol. Hormones that provide a burst of energy see off the hormones associated with depression, so to speak. From a psychological perspective too, the appeal of anxiety aggression is easy to understand. If only for a short time, you trade powerlessness for a sense of power which can even be compounded by an element of vengeance: the chance to inflict on others the same feeling that plagued you only moments before.

In human interaction, anxiety aggression is far more common than predator aggression. Interesting cases can be found in many classical psychiatric studies, such as the analysis that Robert Gaupp and his students at the University of Tübingen made of the massacre committed by Ernst August Wagner, a head teacher with a sombre disposition, angular eyebrows and a classic curled moustache. Extravagant facial hair aside, Wagner appeared to be a thoughtful, rational man; a pillar of the community. But on the morning of 4 September 1913, he stabbed his wife and four children to death. He then travelled to a nearby village where he set fire to a number of buildings and went on a shooting spree, killing nine people and injuring eleven others. Newspaper reports variously dismissed Wagner as being of unsound mind or the devil incarnate. However, an extensive and probing investigation revealed Wagner's motive to be social anxiety. He had a deep-seated fear of people finding out that he masturbated compulsively, harboured homosexual desires, and had sodomised an unspecified animal in the summer of 1901. (You might think that masturbation and homosexuality were the least of his worries in the light of sodomising livestock, but these were different times.) He killed his wife for fear she would leave him if she learned of his behaviour. He killed his children for fear they had inherited his deviant tendencies. And he killed the rest of his victims for fear they might speak out about his behaviour. Ernst August Wagner killed out of shame and fear. His social anxieties became more than he could bear, with this horrific killing spree as a result.

Of course, Wagner was a deeply disturbed individual. His underlying fear of social exposure is something we are all familiar with, but what pushed him over the edge and sparked the psychotic reasoning that moved him to murder was his inability to temper his fear. As Wagner's diary reveals, he felt so beleaguered that he had no choice but to act. It was almost the urge of a cornered animal. Instead of maintaining his defensive façade (which no one had even recognised as such), he acted on an aggressive imperative with gruesome and excessive results. Wagner ended up in an asylum in Winnenthal, where he lived on for many years and even wrote a number of plays.

More recent history is also littered with examples of anxiety aggression. When we look at the more infamous terrorist killings of years gone by, fear repeatedly emerges as the motive. The sense of being threatened appears to play a crucial role in the radicalisation of individuals who, turning their back on society, contemplate committing what they see as a major act of corrective violence.

Fear of the "great replacement" led Anders Breivik to kill seventy-seven innocent people in 2011. Breivik confessed his crime almost immediately, stating that his intention had been to save Norway and the rest of Europe from being overrun by Muslims. Shortly before the start of his trial, Breivik read out a statement calling for his release as a hero who had prevented cultural genocide by launching a "pre-emptive attack against traitors".

Fear of immigration and job losses led Patrick Wood Crusius to shoot twenty-three people at a Walmart store in El Paso, Texas, on 3 August, 2019. Before the killings, a manifesto later attributed to Crusius was posted online, railing against the influence of evil multinationals seeking to cut costs by bringing in cheap migrant labour and embracing automation. Given the high standard of living Americans enjoy, the manifesto argues, these widespread practices will not change any time soon. This leads the writer to reach a bizarre conclusion: "The next logical step is to decrease the number of people in America." Here, a fateful disconnect occurs between the apparent trigger for Crusius's fears – a largely automated society in which major corporations rule the roost: a fear based in reality – and his course of action, which was not directed at multinationals or advocates of automation but at innocent people, almost all of them from the Latino community. A biologist might see this as "redirected behaviour": a conflicted animal directing its hostility at a third participant that has nothing to do with the conflict, purely because they present a readily available outlet for anxiety aggression.

Of course, there are numerous reasons – personal and societal – that may lead people to disengage from the wider community and plot a "corrective" act of violence. Neither Breivik nor Crusius was found to be of unsound mind. Unlike Wagner, their fear was not delusional. Their radicalisation was gradual. But going by their own statements, the fear of a perceived external threat was consistently present at the root of that twisted process. It is also worth noting that anxiety aggression does not always lead to a single, all-encompassing destructive act. Other fears have seen a resurgence in recent years (in conspiracy theories such as QAnon), fears that centre on the power of perverse elites and the supposed global dominance of a powerful Jewish lobby. But while these notions have entered the worldview of large groups of people, they have yet to prompt a murderous act of terror, though some would argue that the storming of the US Capitol fits that description.

Such acts of terror are extreme outbursts, often allied to a more widely shared, socially accepted rhetoric which some politicians choose to amplify rather than tone down. In ancient Greece,

Aristotle formulated the three conditions a political message needs to meet in order to successfully capitalise on people's fears. First, a politician has to warn of an event or development (usually an invasion by "barbarians") that threatens the survival of the group. Second, they should give the impression that this threat is imminent. Third, they must engender a sense that it may already be too late, that urgent action is needed to ensure survival. It should come as no surprise to see these points recurring again and again in political speeches.

Radicalisation, both individual and collective, is a fascinating process but it lies beyond the scope of my search. The point I am making is that, for different reasons and in different ways, fear can play a crucial role on the path to violence.

\*

Sitting in my boyhood bedroom, I start organising my old Batman comics, chronologically and then thematically. One major difference between violent superheroes and largely non-violent mortals is that superheroes have a clear-cut origin story, as it is known in comic-book parlance. They come complete with a well-rounded background – a nurture narrative – that neatly joins the dots between the events from their past and who they have become; a little short on nuance and ambiguity, and just grotesque enough. A superhero could tell their origin story a hundred times and every time it would be identical and strike exactly the same chord with us. Short of fibbing, we mortals will always be denied this luxury. Not that this stops us trying to cobble together a narrative that is more or less coherent, though we are constantly having to reshape and reinterpret, never arriving at a final version. Which events do we select as illustrative, symbolic or even defining? Which do we leave out altogether? Who do we cast as friends, who are our enemies? There is no scriptwriter or director on hand to help us.

The deeper reasons for my stormy, anxious childhood continue to elude me. I know there was an unpredictable side to the love I experienced in this house where I grew up. But whether that was down to the vagaries of my father's character or my own anxious predisposition (which can be traced back through my family history on my mother's side) ... who's to say? Nurture narratives are so personal and unique that they pale in comparison to the seemingly unambiguous, scientific heft of the statistics that demonstrate the influence of nature. To my mind, that imbalance is unjustified.

I flip open the old copy of *Aloha* one more time, and reread the editorial by A.J. Heerma van Voss. "For children of his generation, there will no longer be any reason to want to run away from home [...] It is important that he forms attachments to as many people as possible."

Almost ready to leave my childhood home behind, I open one more book: a 1994 anthology of poetry selected by prominent female figures of the time. It falls open at the poem "My Son" by Anna Enquist.

> My son storms through the house
> a rumble on the stairs. He is
> a motor unto himself. The song
> that lives in him escapes him
> sometimes. I hear him singing
> in the hallway and keep quiet.
>
> At night he is afraid, he doubts
> himself, us, and the world.
> I put my arm around him
> and, without speaking, haze away
> war and childhood cancer
> my own death, the monster of time.
>
> I lie to him and save him
> until we sleep in shared and stolen safety.

Below the poem is a commentary written by my mother, who selected it. Twenty years after my father speculated about the son he might one day have, she looked back on my childhood: "This poem reminds me so much of my elder son. The starkness of the contrast between the vitality, noise and constant activity – *a rumble on the stairs, a motor unto himself* – and the fears, doubts, tears and feeling small. [. . .] What I find comforting about this poem is the protection it offers, keeping trouble at bay, the disasters we all fear, grown-ups as well as children. Brushing all those fears aside for a while. Children have so many fears: of death, illness, separation, war. And those fears emerge at night. In the daytime they play, their minds are occupied. But at night, when they can't sleep, the fears come. The image Enquist conjures up is not one of security, peace and calm, but of a very insecure world: *stolen safety*."

I leave my parents' home, that sanctuary of stolen safety, and step back into the real world, peopled by others, strangers with life stories I can only guess at. Cyclists whizz past, car horns blare, faces swim in and out of my peripheral vision. But many of these life stories have a common element, I realise, as I head for the station. And that element is fear.

In the twentieth century, fear underwent a significant trans-formation: from a concept with philosophical resonance, offering scope for introspection and personal exploration, it became a purely medical matter. This was a transformation on a vast scale. Our ongoing fears morphed into the condition we know today as anxiety disorder. A shift that has had a huge impact on the daily reality of millions of people, who suddenly found themselves suffering from an illness.

# 7

## *Birth of an Illness*

The train glides through the Dutchest of landscapes – flat pastures dotted with motionless cows and framed by dark-water ditches. I knock back my third coffee of the day after another trying night, thick with memories that smouldered like nightmares. My destination is the leafy town of Driebergen, where a landmark conference of the ADF is being held – one of the world's first foundations for people living with anxiety, phobias and compulsive behaviour. When it began, the foundation was little more than a social club, the initiative of one woman battling her own fears. Marina de Wolf-Ferdinandusse was born in 1924, and if anyone's life can attest to the shape-shifting nature of fear in the twentieth century, it is hers.

The story of her fears begins in 1962, with a fateful trip to visit friends. Husband Hans – breadwinner and factory foreman – had decided it was time she got out of the house for a change. Hans and Marina had met through the Resistance and married shortly after the Second World War. In the Nazi-occupied Netherlands, Marina had helped Jews go into hiding and would always be haunted by the memory of those who did not survive. The early sixties was a tough time for Marina. She underwent a series of operations on her jaw and had to tend to her ailing mother, who had suffered a heart attack. She and Hans moved house twice and she gave birth to two daughters, from whom she contracted chicken pox. By 1962, she was exhausted. For weeks, she had been feeling listless, queasy, dizzy. Her knees often seemed to buckle under her. Kierkegaard wrote that fear, if unrecognised, goes underground and waits for the moment when you are vulnerable: a time of crisis, when certainties have fallen away and all your reserves are gone. That's how it was for Marina.

As she and Hans sat chatting with their friends, the conversation turned to physical frailty and mortality; a number of the friends' relatives were struggling to cope with one illness or another. Marina was deeply affected by what she heard. "From one minute to the next, I began to feel terribly ill," she later described. "I couldn't breathe, my heart was pounding, the whole room started spinning." A panic attack, at a time when the term had yet to be coined. Her friends invited her to lie down on the couch and fetched her a blanket, but nothing could stop her shaking. The local GP was summoned and, when he was unable to find the cause, Marina was rushed to hospital and held overnight. The next day, the doctor assured her that two weeks of bed rest was all she needed. He was wrong.

In her own words, Marina had "come down with something" and that something showed no sign of letting up. Every time she stepped outside, she began to hyperventilate. Before long, she hardly dared to get up and would spend all day in bed or lying on the couch. It was the start of a tortuous journey that took her to neurologists, internists and other specialists. She ended up in psychoanalysis with a therapist who mostly wanted to talk about the war. She talked four days a week for eighteen months and then she stopped. Marina de Wolf-Ferdinandusse had said all there was to say.

But the *something* remained. From 1962 to 1970, she barely left the house. Other people fetched her groceries. She had new clothes delivered and sent back anything that didn't fit. If there was anything *actually* wrong with her, her friends said, surely the doctor would have found it by now. They hinted that if she really wanted to get better, she would have shaken this thing a long time ago. Marina was left feeling furious, lonely, desperate. And if she was feeling this way, she reasoned, there must be others with similar experiences. The medical profession had little to offer. Anxiety, phobias and other mental health problems were not yet part of the medical curriculum, so there was next to no chance of a GP recognising the plight of someone with anxiety.

Yet by the end of the 1960s, Marina had found a way to expand her world. She had become fascinated by a British organisation called The Open Door, the first association in the world to focus on phobias. It was founded in 1966 by Alice Neville, a woman who had suffered from severe anxiety since the aerial bombardments that had pounded wartime London during the Blitz: flashing lights, wailing sirens, the drone of bombers overhead, explosion after explosion. Through an acquaintance, Alice found work as a secretary at MI6. Her fears intensified until they felt like a hand tightening around her throat. On the bus into London one day, she went weak at the knees and began to hyperventilate. It was the start of a process that eventually led her to found The Open Door, convinced that she had to overcome this problem before it overcame her.

Marina de Wolf-Ferdinandusse identified so much with Alice – her sensitivities, her wartime panic, the implosion of her social life – that she followed in her footsteps and founded the Dutch Phobia Association in 1968. Both Alice and Marina were way ahead of their time. The Anxiety Disorders Association of America, for example, was only set up in 1980. On 1 March, 1969, the first edition of *The Phobia Vizier* was published: the bimonthly club magazine, which Marina "knocked together" (her words) at the kitchen table, sipping a neglected cup of lukewarm tea. Each year at Christmas, her husband Hans would write a reflective piece, solidly Christian in tone. Marina's forewords took the form of personal accounts that provide a unique picture of how the Netherlands and the rest of Europe were changing between 1968 and 1997: thirty years in which the popular perception of anxiety transformed and treatments evolved, with all that this entailed.

Soon after the club was founded, Marina's instinct about the widespread nature of fear was proved right. The readers' letters published during the first years of her magazine constituted a collective sigh of relief. "Every town, every village," she wrote in those early days, "is home to one or more phobia sufferers. Cries for help have reached us from all parts of the country." An initial membership of five shot up to one thousand in a matter of months and kept on growing. These were people whose daily lives were severely disrupted by their fears; some had not left the house for years, lives confined to a few dozen square metres. People who were afraid of trembling or blushing, of illness or incontinence, of cancer, animals, children, Christmas trees. As strange as some of these phobias sound, they can always be traced back to objects or phenomena that have been a threat to survival in the course of human history: trees can fall on you, animals bite, unaccepted social behaviour can lead to rejection by the group. Almost everyone who confided in Marina said they found it very hard to talk about their fears with their loved ones. Some who did described the risks of talking too much: marriages that were hollowed out, the firmest of friendships derailed. Directly or indirectly, fear always led to a profound sense of loneliness. Marina took to calling the members her "fellow fearties".

Most of those fearties were women and, strikingly, this is still the case. To this day, women are one and a half times more likely to be diagnosed with an anxiety disorder than men, regardless of age group. A 2014 study conducted by Florida State University bio-medical scientist Mohamed Kabbaj concluded that testosterone – a hormone generally present at far higher levels in men than in women – might function as a neurological buffer against anxiety.

Meanwhile, the hormones oestrogen and progesterone – which women generally have more of than do men – are thought to make habituation to threatening situations more difficult, even when a threat has been shown not to be genuine. But social factors are seen to be equally important. Women may experience greater pressures in their everyday lives than men, or perhaps they traditionally feel freer, or even duty bound, to express the anxiety they feel. No-one really knows and very little research has been done, presumably for fear of becoming entangled in a thorny gender debate. The only researcher to make a serious attempt to explain the difference between men and women with respect to one particular fear was sociologist Abram de Swaan (the same sociologist who advised my mother to try psycho-analysis). De Swaan argued that the lifting of stringent restrictions on the mobility of well-to-do European women in the nineteenth century led to a new condition. As these restrictions were removed, the first cases of *Platzschwindel* (literally "square dizziness" – square as in a large, open public place) began to appear in psychiatric literature, a term later replaced by the more stylish-sounding "ago-raphobia". What in the nineteenth century had been a matter of desirably restrained behaviour – not venturing into the streets where one might mix with the lower classes – rapidly became a neurotic condition at the beginning of the twentieth century. It is an appealing theory, albeit one that is hard to either confirm or debunk.

In the association's infancy, Marina saw it as her goal to offer the lonely and the outcast a sense of connection. Wary of elaborate programmes and outspoken principles, she saw her initiative as "a contact agency" that provided messages of support and practical tips, such as how to fold a facemask to counter hyperventilation. But Marina's main aim was to bring her fellow fearties under the care of the right doctors. No mean feat in 1968, when the Nether-lands averaged a mere one and a half therapists per province. In the far north and Zeeland in the south, it was practically impossible to find professional help. And pills? They were "poison for the nervous system", as one member wrote in 1969.

When the association marked its tenth anniversary in 1978, Marina paused to reflect. "It's incredible to think how much has changed in the course of a decade. When the club started, there were only twenty therapists in the entire country . . . And just look at the options available today. Many psychologists have even gone on to specialise in particular fears." In other words, society was changing and fear was fast becoming a legitimate clinical condition for which serious treatments were being developed. In the 1970s, people mainly put their faith in psychotherapy, in talking. Psychotherapists operated on the assumption that symptoms of anxiety were non-specific expressions of something deeper, something that had to be coaxed to the surface through conversation or it would go on to manifest itself in other, more destructive ways. But Marina had her reservations. She had always been more interested in solutions than causes, favouring practical interventions such as relaxation techniques, reading, talking on the phone, arts and crafts, anything to steer attention away from the anxiety itself. That said, she was by no means part of the anti-authoritarian backlash at the time, neatly illustrated by one member's insistence on writing the word "psychiatrist" as "psyche-hater-ist". At the heart of the anti-psychiatry movement that emerged in the 1960s was the conviction that society, not the patient, was sick. To Marina, this was little more than a clever play on words that ultimately benefited no-one.

As healthcare underwent a professional transformation in the 1970s, Marina's self-professed contact agency was also evolving. In 1978, it went from being an association to a foundation in a bid to do more for those who were struggling to afford treatment. Instead of simply connecting the lonely, Marina became a pivotal figure with far-reaching influence and the knowledge to guide her fellow fearties through the confusing, expanding and ever-changing world of treatment. She protected them from quacks, healers, magnetisers, reincarnation therapists and all manner of charlatans who took their money and left them feeling even more alone and frustrated. Mulling all this over on the train, I catch myself wishing I could have got to know Marina personally. But knowing all this about her comes a close second.

The medical-scientific underpinning of Marina's pragmatic approach did not surface until the 1980s, when cognitive behavioural therapy (CBT) came along. This theory explained fears as misguided beliefs and forms of behaviour, instead of past problems as yet unprocessed. "As a fearty," she said in 1976, "you have learned an incorrect pattern of behaviour. And so it has to be unlearned."

The notion that fear is a false belief goes back millennia. According to the Roman philosopher, orator and politician Cicero, fear is a belief about an impending evil that we think we cannot handle. The main difference between fear and sorrow, he argued, is that fear is caused by something in the future and sorrow by something in the past. Fear and sorrow arise from our belief that the threats and dangers in the world are substantial and real. But Cicero insists that this is not the case. All dangers and all pleasures are transient. The appropriate response is to keep things in perspective and to be moderate and stoic at all times. (Yes, good old stoicism!) Cicero was strongly influenced by the Stoics, who advocated being imperturbable in the face of whatever life throws at us. But he also heeded Epicurus, who noted that even wealthy rulers who, on the face of it had nothing to fear, were often beset by fears and anxiety. This led Epicurus to formulate a philosophical ideal, which he believed we should all strive to attain: *ataraxia*, a mind free from worry. Along similar lines, the Roman philosopher Seneca later asserted that *tranquillitas animi* (peace of mind) is by far the most important quality in life. His advice was to detach ourselves from our useless fears, perhaps the most useless of all being fear of death. The first step, Seneca, argues is to abandon all hope: "Cease to hope . . . and you will cease to fear . . . Just as the same chain fastens the prisoner and the soldier who guards him, so hope and fear, dissimilar as they are, keep step together; fear follows hope."

Another Stoic, the Greek philosopher Epictetus, who had been born into slavery, believed it was not the world that made us unhappy, but our conceptions of the world. In his discourse "Of Anxiety" he writes "When I see any one anxious, I say, 'what does this man want?' Unless he wanted something or other not in his own power, how could he still be anxious? A musician, for instance, feels no anxiety while he is singing by himself; but when he appears upon the stage he does, even if his voice be ever so good, or he plays ever so well. For what he wishes is not only to sing well, but likewise to gain applause. But this is not in his own power." Epictetus argued that you could face down your fears by reasoning logically and thinking about what you can and cannot affect, views that would recur in a slightly modified form in the work of the seventeenth-century Dutch philosopher Baruch Spinoza, who argued that fear was essentially non-logical. In brief, Spinoza's hyper-rational view of fear states that if you cannot influence something, there is no point in being afraid of it; after all, you're powerless. And if you *can* influence something, then what is the point in being afraid when you can work to change it? Conclusion: it never makes sense to be afraid. As you may have gathered, Spinoza's ideal human was a purely rational being.

The similarities between these centuries-old notions and the principles of cognitive behavioural therapy are striking. CBT is one of the most widely deployed approaches to tackling anxiety. It teaches you to think differently (change your cognitions) about your fears, rather than running away from them or countering them with medication. Meanwhile the Stoic idea of living in the moment has been given a remarkable new lease of life as the motto of countless mindfulness retreats.

Ancient philosophers aside, it took a nine-month-old baby boy weighing twenty-one pounds to revive the idea of fear as a mistaken belief. Little Albert was his name. Born in the United States in

1919, he would become the subject of an experiment devised and described by John Watson, a beady-eyed psychologist with a tight-lipped smile. Little Albert was anything but anxious. He would happily pet all kinds of animals and even the sight of a rat failed to startle him. But for some reason, the sound of a gong sent him into a panic. This gave Watson an idea: what if someone were to strike a gong whenever Albert held out his chubby little hand to a rat? This only had to be repeated seven times to saddle the boy with the beginnings of a phobia: once the association had been established, he would recoil on seeing a rat even if the gong was not sounded. Not only that, but the same anxious response was soon triggered by dogs, rabbits and even inanimate furry objects. Watson had demonstrated that it was possible to influence the development of fears. And if fear could be learned, as Little Albert had shown, Watson and the therapists who came after him concluded that it could also be unlearned.

A second key figure in the history of this theory is the psychiatrist, psychoanalyst and war veteran Aaron T. Beck. He used word association when working with his patients and noticed that they kept coming back to the same thoughts, associations that were a torment to them rather than a help. Beck labelled them "automatic thoughts". In the early 1970s, he designed a method to build his patients' resilience to these automatic thoughts, and cognitive behavioural therapy was born. The key to CBT was not to avoid your fears. The technical term for this pragmatic approach was "exposure": exposing yourself to whatever frightens you enables you to learn that the fear is unfounded. Don't be afraid of fear itself: breathe calmly and whatever you do, don't succumb to the idea that you are going mad. People with agoraphobia were encouraged to go outside and walk a little further each day, from one lamp post to the next, reclaiming neutral terrain one patch at a time; it was all about taking that first step. In a similar vein, Marina advised people to buy a car – "a house on wheels" she called it – so that they could always get away under their own steam. This could give them something to hold on to, that little bit of control. And otherwise they should get a dog to help them through the day. Dogs, she said, were "medicine on legs".

Marina's almost maternal care for her fellow fearties was her salvation, but it also left her vulnerable. In the 1970s, she became anxiety personified. Her regular TV appearances invariably prompted hundreds of letters, all of which she answered personally. For much of the day, her dining table was a postal depot. The phone rang day and night, often to the annoyance of the children. Privacy became a thing of the past: her fearties always came first. The pressure was building and something had to give. One day, when Hans was driving Marina to her therapist, their dark-blue Chevrolet Impala ran into a traffic jam and Marina had a full-blown panic attack. Hans responded by pulling over, slamming the gear stick into reverse and barrelling backwards down the hard shoulder to the nearest exit. They laughed about it later, but the lesson was clear: Marina would never completely overcome her anxious sensibilities. Very occasionally, I see something of myself and D. in Hans and Marina's relationship: a blend of love and incomprehension, the best of intentions undermined by helplessness.

It was only when Hans developed cancer and she had to visit him in hospital that Marina ventured out into the world. "It hit me one day when I had to drive sixty miles," she said. "Three miles had been my absolute limit. But I did it, without thinking twice." For the first time she felt that she had "conquered" her agoraphobia, for as long as it lasted. Conquer: a word that suited Marina down to the ground.

The realisation that not everyone with the same struggle had the same genetic armoury at their disposal did not sit well with Marina's way of thinking. At a meeting in May 1972, when someone in the audience asked if phobias were hereditary, she answered with an unequivocal "No!" It was a view she regularly aired in her newsletter. She recognised that anxiety, like many other forms of mental illness, tends to run in families, but put this down to how those families handled their fears: if your mother or brother is clearly terrified of birds, it's only a matter of time before you start scanning the skies for danger too. As Marina saw it, anxious behaviour was contagious.

In the early 1980s, her forewords became more professional in tone, more business-like; a change that coincided with a significant development in the medical world. In 1980, "anxiety disorder" was included as a condition in the third edition of the DSM, the official medical reference work on mental health issues. Excessive anxiety had gained official recognition as an illness. It is also worth noting what anxiety lost in that process: its status as a bodily imbalance (Hippocrates), a misguided attitude to life (the Stoics) and a philosophical problem (Kierkegaard). From that day forth, anxiety was a brain-based disorder. To understand how we reached this point in the 1980s, it makes sense to zoom out and consider the route that took us there.

My train pulls into Utrecht and I find my way to the local bus that will take me on to Driebergen. Hurried steps all around me, paper cups discarded and trampled underfoot: rush hour. Time to ease away from the crowds and head back to the nineteenth century, to the University of Tartu on the banks of the Emajõgi, the river that threads together the largest lakes in Estonia. Back then, this small Baltic state was part of the Russian Empire and the university's clinic was under the charge of a German psychiatrist named Emil Kraepelin. He may well have been the first to open Pandora's box. The first, but certainly not the last.

# 8

## *Pandora's Boxes*

As I board the bus to the conference organised by Marina's foundation, I take out my phone and swipe through some photos of the distinguished professor and his feather duster of a moustache. In many ways, Emil Kraepelin can be considered the anti-Freud. He was not especially interested in a patient's hidden story, in the dark recesses of their being. His primary concern was the body, its genetic make-up, its biology: any aspect that could be measured, in line with the scientific dictates of the Enlightenment. Frustrated by the outcomes of his laboratory studies, which had been a moderate success at best, he focused on what would go on to become the core of his doctrine: detailed patient histories or *Zählkarte* as he called them. In these *Zählkarte*, essentially the precursors of our modern medical records, Kraepelin noted every change, however small, in the behaviour of his patients.

Towards the end of the nineteenth century, after years of research, he felt ready to share his new classification of mental illness with the world. He was in a position, he said, to distinguish between a number of archetypes of mental illness. These included categories that can be seen as early delineations of what we now call schizophrenia and bipolar disorder. Kraepelin referred to the traditional classification as "symptomatic" and his own approach as "clinical". But this clinical approach required the thorough and systematic study of a large number of cases, not least because he believed that all the symptoms of one disease were also present in others. Kraepelin's focus was not on the symptoms themselves, but on the pattern they formed, a pattern that varied with each condition. He saw anxiety as a central deregulation of the body, a symptom that could be detected in any pattern, and which therefore did not constitute a separate medical category. Kraepelin was convinced that every mental affliction was rooted in the brain or the genes – human biology, in other words. He demonstrated this through comparative studies: schizophrenics tended to come from families where schizophrenia was more prevalent, while people with a bipolar disorder also had a relatively high number of family members who suffered from mania or depression.

We have the US Armed Forces and the Second World War to thank for bringing Kraepelin's scientific legacy to the masses. The vast deployment of troops during the war gave the US government cause for reflection. Traditional psychiatric methods were simply too time-consuming to facilitate the diagnosis and treatment of traumatised soldiers on such a large scale. It was time to remove mental illness from the realm of grand theories dreamed up by lone scholars and to favour a more scientific approach that could be used by any doctor: one that was measurable, objective, clear and widely applicable. A committee headed by psychiatrist and military man Brigadier General William C. Menninger therefore devised a new classification scheme, bearing Kraepelin's categories in mind. Dubbed "Medical 203", it was adopted by the Navy, the Army, and veterans' organisations with only a few minor adjustments. In 1949, the World Health Organization added some passages relating specifically to mental illness. However, a streamlined approach for the average American was still a long way off in a country where every hospital worked according to its own system. In the resulting disarray, the call for a single standardised method grew louder by the day. Medical 203 was seen as the answer, and in 1951, after a brief round of editing, a modified version of a classification system originally conceived to process as many military personnel as possible as quickly as possible was published as the *Diagnostic and Statistical Manual of Mental Disorders*, soon shortened to DSM.

The first edition, DSM I, was published in 1952. This 130-page document listed 106 mental illnesses, including homosexuality (classified as a sociopathic personality disorder). It was structured along the same lines as Medical 203 and many passages were copied verbatim. In DSM I, anxiety was one of the main features of all neurotic disorders, a "signal" that the patient was unconsciously battling unresolved inner conflicts. This would either give rise to a "fear response" or, if it centred on a particular object or situation, to a "phobic reaction". Vintage Freud, in other words.

DSM II, published in 1968, gave more prominence to neurosis as a category and to anxiety as the main feature of neurosis. By this time, anxiety and neurosis had become virtually synonymous. The compilers of DSM II distinguished between an anxiety neurosis characterised by general worry and panic, a phobic neurosis, an obsessive-compulsive neurosis (what we now call obsessive-compulsive disorder or OCD) and a depressive neurosis.

In 1980, DSM III saw the light of day and constituted a radical departure from its predecessors, thanks to not only its format but also the revolutionary way it came about. In its third incarnation, the manual had given anxiety a place of its own, reborn as a stand-alone disorder, out from the shadow of neurosis. This decoupling of anxiety and neurosis effectively wrested anxiety from the grip of the Freudians and this was of huge importance to Marina, who had no truck with Freud and his wild theories and was frankly embarrassed by their sexual overtones and obsession with castration. DSM III gave Marina confirmation of what she had known for a long time: she had not been exaggerating or overstating her case. Anxiety was an "actual illness". DSM III divided anxiety disorders into phobias and anxiety states. Phobias were subdivided into agoraphobia, social phobia and phobias of objects. Agoraphobia and fear of blushing, for example, were seen as having a significant social component in that they are not so much about open spaces or blushing in themselves as they are about negative exposure to the gaze of others. Strictly speaking, they are about fear of fear. The "anxiety states" were subdivided into panic disorder, generalised anxiety disorder, obsessive-compulsive disorder and post-traumatic stress syndrome. The basis on which these particular disorders were divided up brings us to some unsettling revelations about how DSM III took shape.

The bus picks up speed and I leave the city behind, trading urban shrubbery for the leafy lanes of suburbia. Nondescript terraces make way for sequestered villas.

The nature of DSM III cannot be fully understood without addressing the work of US psychiatrist Donald F. Klein. When he passed away in 2019, his obituary referred to him as "the father of psychopharmacology". In the 1950s, Klein discovered that a certain drug, imipramine, blocked panic attacks in people with agoraphobia but not in people with chronic anxiety or other types of phobia. One patient in particular, who ran to the nurses' desk in panic every few hours because he thought he was dying, improved greatly on imipramine. That is, his feelings of anxiety barely diminished but their physical manifestation in the form of panic all but disappeared. This pharmacological difference led Klein to infer that panic and anxiety must be different syndromes, as opposed to a panic attack being seen as an acute, exacerbated expression of chronic anxiety. This may seem like a minor observation, but in fact it represents a fundamental reversal of how research into illnesses had always been conducted. Instead of the illness defining the drug, the drug had come to define the illness. About this turnaround, British psychoanalyst Darian Leader writes that "rather than seeing the drug as key to the lock of the illness, the illness was defined as whatever would fit that key, rather like Cinderella's slipper."

Although Klein's findings were consistently criticised from a scientific standpoint, pharmaceutical companies smelled an opportunity. The 1960s and 1970s saw an unstoppable wave of pharmacological research, studies that required an increasingly precise set of criteria and definitions based on outward manifestations and symptoms. When, in the early 1970s, it became clear that the DSM was to be revised a second time, these companies asserted their influence. Behind closed doors at the Hilton Hotel in St. Louis, Missouri, a task force of psychiatrists brought together in 1974 discussed which syndromes would be defined in DSM III. Psychoanalysts and psychologists were excluded from these discussions as much as possible, signalling a crucial power shift at a pivotal moment: the moment when our view of anxiety was about to be defined for years to come.

Psychiatrist David Sheehan, who attended as a consultant, remembers the occasion well. The task force discussed Klein's work for a while before determining that panic disorder was a legitimate illness. "And then the wine flowed some more, and the psychiatrists around the dinner table started talking about one of their colleagues who didn't suffer from panic attacks but who worried all the time. How would we classify him? He's just sort of *generally* anxious. Hey, how about 'generalized anxiety disorder'? And then they toasted the christening of the disease with the next bottle of wine. And then for the next thirty years the world collected data on it." Others present went on to describe the underlying research as "a hodgepodge – scattered, inconsistent and ambiguous". Sometimes the advocate of a particular "condition" based their argument on dealings with a single patient. Supposed experts advocated "diseases" such as "chronic complaint disorder", with symptoms that covered whining about anything from the weather to taxes and last night's track results, and answering the question "How are you?" by sighing "Oy vay, don't ask".

"We thrashed it out, basically," another person involved recalls. "We had a three-hour argument. There would be about twelve people sitting down at a table, usually there was a chairperson and there was somebody taking notes [...] If people were still divided, the matter would eventually be decided by a vote." This usually meant a show of hands. "Our team was certainly not typical of the psychiatry community," Robert Spitzer, the head of the task force, said in an interview in 2012. "DSM III [...] allowed a small group with a particular viewpoint to take over psychiatry and change it in a fundamental way. [...] It was a revolution [...] We took over because we had the power." And so it came to pass that a few dozen people influenced the fate of tens of millions. Simply because they could.

Unfortunately for us, the task force members signed an agreement that prohibited them from publicly talking about what went on at these meetings. The public did not receive full disclosure until a few years ago, when the archives of the American Psychiatric Association were opened. They revealed that a large proportion of the DSM III researchers had contracts with one of the pharmaceutical companies with a financial interest in which disorders received official status. An officially recognised condition would effectively create a gap in the market, an opportunity to make billions in profits. Of the researchers reportedly involved in drawing up DSM IV (1994), as many as 56 per cent were thought to have financial ties with the pharmaceutical industry.

Unsurprisingly, this interference has resulted in each new edition of the DSM specifying more disorders than its predecessor. DSM III contained about three times as many as DSM I, and featured such new gems as "caffeine intoxication disorder", "mathematics disorder" and "frotteurism" (seeking arousal by illicitly rubbing up against someone). Pathological labels were also conferred on character traits such as shyness, which became "avoidant personality disorder" or "social anxiety disorder". On a positive note, DSM III no longer classified homosexuality as a mental illness.

In contrast to DSM I, a humble ring-bound affair, DSM III

was a hefty and compelling tome. This once slimline framework had been bulked up into a supposedly comprehensive catalogue that would go on to have an unprecedented impact on medical practice. A condition that did not feature in the catalogue was seldom acknowledged by the medical community, and insurers were seldom prepared to cover the cost of treating such "spurious" conditions. Compare DSM IV to the document at the root of it all – the original Medical 203 – and the number of psychiatric diagnoses is a staggering 800 per cent higher. DSM V, the edition in use since 2013, contains even more conditions. The human tendency to expand the number of medical labels and syndromes has long been a cause for concern, but in recent decades it has really hit its stride. This point was neatly made by psychologist Paul Verhaeghe when he proposed that Mania Diagnostica Activa (MDA) – or diagnosis mania – be granted official DSM recognition.

Roughly from the start of the 1960s, science and psychiatry began to develop side by side at an unprecedented rate, a dynamic that dovetailed seamlessly with the capitalist faith in market forces: the psychopharmaceutical multinational was born. At the same time, alternative points of view were becoming increasingly thin on the ground. And at a crucial juncture, without explicit permission, a global system emerged in which anxiety (and many other mental states) were almost automatically categorised as an illness. Let's call this system the DSM regime, after the reference work at its core.

Under the DSM regime, the main currency consists of semi-coincidental labels generated by conversations between people whose position as regards the link between psychiatry and phar-maceuticals was not exactly neutral. Diagnoses were thrashed out by "a bunch of guys sitting at a table". Studies showing that an estimated 25 per cent of long-term psychiatric patients are living with the consequences of an incorrect or outdated label have done little to change this situation.

None of the dozens of doctors I spoke to for this book were aware of the dubious genesis of the supposedly objective instrument that is so central to their work. Some believe they are at the mercy of what they see as a perverse system. Many recognise the flawed nature of this DSM regime, which has no single ruler but millions of slaves with no choice but to practise according to its dictates or risk losing their prestige, their connections within the healthcare system and perhaps even their medical licence.

The problem is not the fact that the DSM exists. As a guide, it has also brought many benefits. It decreases the likelihood of a mental health problem going undetected. It is a safeguard against healthy people ending up in an institution, as was – and sometimes still is – the case in totalitarian regimes. And of course, psychiatry as it is practised has more to offer than the DSM alone. But we now face the widespread and perhaps insoluble problem that there is no longer an alternative outside the DSM, nor is there any immediate prospect of one in societies where market principles have become so deeply embedded in healthcare institutions, where so much research is sponsored by pharmaceutical companies, and where time and money are always mentioned in the same breath.

The friendly, perhaps even amorous, relationship between the healthcare sector and pharmaceutical companies continues to this day: expenses-paid trips in exchange for promoting a particular drug, conferring corporate-sponsored academic chairs on psychiatrists who are "good for business", boosting the budgets for certain avenues of research. But more subtle forms of influence also prevail, like nudging psychiatrists towards a slight preference for a particular drug knowing it will lead to sizeable profits. Especially in the United States, the world's largest psychopharmaceuticals market, where such practices are a regular occurrence.

In cases where pharmaceutical companies are suspected of directly bribing insurers or members of the medical profession, major lawsuits are sometimes filed. But often corporate influence is more nebulous, as in the case of industry-sponsored "ambassadors" or "key opinion leaders". Although people in these roles may not have a direct relationship with patients, they can still entice an insurer or treating physician to opt for a particular drug. Even a relatively small market like the Netherlands is not immune to such practices. The late Louis Tas, a prominent psychiatrist in his day, lamented the fact that his beloved profession was being "held hostage by the pharmaceutical industry". Fellow psychiatrist Witte Hoogendijk, while acknowledging that such practices are common, argued that the blame should not be placed entirely at the door of the multinationals. "You could say that the pharmaceutical industry is the one sincere party in the medical world. They simply want to make as much profit as possible." That's one way of looking at it.

As I reflect on all this, the bus reaches Driebergen, where Marina lived through the early days of the DSM regime. But before we arrive at our destination, let's take a detour to the Europe of the 1980s, the decade in which I was born.

It was a time of graffiti slogans and Arafat scarves, of an entire generation labelled "lost" as the unemployment rate hovered well above 10 per cent. A time of cultural pessimism and prophecies of doom. In 1986, Reactor 4 at the Chernobyl nuclear power plant exploded in what was then the Ukrainian Soviet Socialist Republic. Terrorism was rife: the IRA, Germany's Baader-Meinhof Gang, Italy's Red Brigades and Basque separatists ETA in Spain. And then there was The Bomb. In the Netherlands, some GPs held a special surgery for patients struggling to cope with their fears of all-out nuclear war. Another group of doctors called on the government to spare its citizens a slow and painful death from radiation poisoning by providing a suicide pill.

Between 1980 (the year anxiety gained official recognition as a disorder) and 1987, the number of people who turned to Marina's foundation for information shot up from seventeen thousand to fifty thousand. Reports of anxiety in children also seemed to be on the rise. "Lately," she wrote in June 1983, "I have been struck by the number of calls I receive from parents worried that what their children are hearing at school is causing them to dwell compulsively on issues like air pollution, pesticides and nuclear waste." It was a time when acid rain and forest dieback were all over the news.

Similar climate fears exist today, of course, often in intensified form. Large numbers of people worldwide suffer from eco woes, so much so that the American Psychiatric Association has recognised "ecoanxiety" as a common condition. In reality, ecoanxiety is a variation on fear of The Bomb: alarm at the prospect of the world's imminent demise combined with a sense of complete powerlessness. In turn, fear of an atomic Armageddon can be seen as an update on the Christian fear of Judgement Day. (You could fill a library with writings on the complex relationship between fear and religion. For now, let's just say that while God is a consolation to some, others are overcome by their fear of Him. The Almighty has the power to exacerbate and to allay our fears.) In 2020, as the Covid crisis took hold, this fear of Judgement Day became disastrously entangled with another primal human fear: that of contamination. Since the dawn of history, we have been aware that an invisible disease, transmitted from one person to another, can bring death. Even a text as ancient as the Babylonian *Epic of Gilgamesh* asserts that the flood is preferable to a deadly contagion. Chinese writings dating from the thirteenth century BCE reveal an awareness of epidemics.

A foray into the newspaper archives confirms the rise of fear in the 1980s. In 2012, the Dutch National Library digitised around 10 million national news articles published between 1618 and 1999 – about 8 per cent of the total volume published in newspapers during that time. A search on the word *angst* (which encompasses both fear and anxiety) reveals a single usage in the seventeenth century, in the *Europische Saterdaegs Courant*. In the eighteenth century, it appeared 394 times. In the nineteenth century, this figure leaped to 70,477. But it was in the twentieth century that fear and anxiety hit the headlines with a vengeance, occurring no less than 610,899 times in news articles. As you might expect, there was a peak between 1930 and 1939, in the lead-up to the Second

World War: 104,558 instances. In the decade after the war, this figure halved, dropping to 39,978 during the 1950s. From there, it began to climb again, with 47,355 mentions between 1960 and 1969 and 59,336 between 1970 and 1979. But the modern decade of fear is really the 1980s, with 81,674 instances between 1980 and 1989: only 20 per cent down on the spike that preceded global conflict. (The 1990s saw this figure decline again, to 52,651.)

"The number of extremely frightened children is on the increase," Marina concluded again in December 1987. "I hear this in what parents tell me. They too will need help in future." It was as if a generation of frightened children was emerging before her very eyes, children who had never known war, yet who derived no sense of security from this fact. When these young fearties grew up, they would go on to form an oddly skittish army, large in number, small in influence. It's an army to which I too belong, born on a January evening in 1986 from the union of a journalist and a sociologist who met at a meeting on mental illness. He remembered her: she was the young woman featured in an article on "new-style divorce" he had edited years before.

Yes, there was the atom bomb. And economic strife. But can anything else account for the massive increase in anxiety that Marina was seeing?

We now know that this increase also relates to what Canadian philosopher Ian Hacking calls "the looping effect". The gist of this idea is that how we describe the world goes on to change the world itself. Hacking based his theory on developments in the 1970s surrounding multiple personality disorder or MPD, often referred to as "split personality". Following several instances of people exhibiting odd behaviour, psychiatrists began to use the label MPD. This led to the disorder being widely reported in the media, which in turn led to a rise in the number of people exhibiting the symptoms that had been reported. Hacking concludes that people had unconsciously taught themselves to exhibit these symptoms, to "take on the role" of someone with MPD, and so were perceived and registered as having the disorder.

The psychology behind this mechanism is not hard to appreciate. Imagine that for years you have been suffering from anxiety, compulsive thoughts, intense feelings of panic or worthlessness. Your behaviour has been qualified as strange, unhealthy, anything but positive. The more you hear these things, the harder it is to talk about how you feel. Until one day you pluck up the courage to go and see a doctor, who has not one but two revelations in store.

First, you are suffering from an officially recognised illness. In other words, you haven't been imagining things. You are not crazy and since you are suffering from a bona fide medical condition, you can't help feeling the way you do. Second, there are drugs available to help you. All you have to do in return is embrace the label you have been given. Unfortunately, that label can only really offer a false sense of security; after all, depression or an anxiety disorder can never be verified using X-rays or blood counts – the diagnosis remains a matter of probability. But as a patient in search of an answer, that's the last thing you want to hear. What makes this so complex is that my symptoms, your symptoms, the symptoms of everyone who leaves the doctor's surgery with a label, are genuine. The existence of the looping effect does not mean that everyone who accepts the associated label is a fraud or an idiot. The problem is that the critical faculties of people enduring real suffering are sometimes compromised by their desperation and their desire to be taken seriously.

I vividly remember my own first brush with the DSM, back in 2013 when I first went to see a psychiatrist. His initial impressions were filed away for posterity: "Well-built young man, friendly. Observant, somewhat reserved. Laughs readily at times. Makes contact easily, but is compulsively preoccupied with fear of failure. His moods fluctuate, but there is a constant undertone of anxiety. Very troubling situation." After listening a while longer, he told me about the existence of the anxiety disorder. So I know it well, that curious sensation, moving in its own way, when you are told there is a group of people to which you might belong. Admittedly, it's not the group you would have signed up to beforehand – not the most prestigious, praiseworthy or sociable group – but those lonely years spent searching for what is troubling you are over. Although labels are nothing more than models devised by human minds, they carry a powerful magnetic charge that bends behaviours and ways of interpreting those behaviours in their direction. The power they demonstrate, the power of simplicity, far outshines other more diffuse explanations, undermined by subjectivity and a lack of professional clout. Sitting opposite the psychiatrist, my panic attacks and all my periods of depression were suddenly rearranged; slotted into a well-rounded model that felt so right, it simply had to be true.

Only, this is a mechanism with a catch. "The problem is that labels can take on a life of their own," Professor Jan Swinkels, psychiatrist at University of Amsterdam Academic Medical Center explains to me in an interview. "Instead of guiding, they lead the way. Twenty years ago, someone who felt anxious might have thought, 'I've been feeling shaky for a while but I can still make a go of things.' Today, the same person thinks 'I have an anxiety disorder. I am ill.' And there are so many advocates for people who are anxious and depressed, well-meaning organisations that have done so much to destigmatise these conditions. . . It's almost impossible for people *not* to start thinking of themselves as 'a suitable case for treatment'. Desperate people are being pushed towards a diagnosis."

Desperate or not, at the time I felt a strong need for clarity. Until that moment, I had looked back on my life as a trail of debris. Things would be fine for a while, but then the anxiety would resurface, gathering momentum until I cracked and slumped into a depression that could last for months. As soon as I got out from under, I would resolve to leave this latest dark episode behind me for ever. Why waste time moping over another chunk of debris when a new phase was dawning, a clean slate? I bought new clothes, made new friends, people who had only ever known this happy and relieved side of me. It was a boom-and-bust life cycle that messed with my memory. Looking at old photos, I caught myself thinking: who is that person? Instead of a single life spanning twenty-five years, it was as if I had lived five separate lives that averaged five years. The psychiatrist helped me see this as an unnecessary and destructive pattern. Each time I came back from the dead and dreamed up a brand-new me, I was denying the underlying truth: the likelihood that what I had just been through would happen all over again. My anxiety, the psychiatrist observed, was almost always triggered when I felt unfairly judged or fell foul of my own unrealistically high expectations, two sets of circumstances that were almost certain to recur with some regularity. The triggers might differ, but the fear was the same. The fear this time around and next time around was the same fear I had experienced when I was six or seven, hearing that plank bridge creak beneath my feet.

The DSM on my psychiatrist's desk was implacable: I exhibited all the symptoms of a panic disorder. After years spent pondering the nature of fear, the answer was handed to me on a plate: it was a neurological and psychological defect. And so, at the age of twenty-six, I entered the world of medicalised anxiety. I accepted the label as if it were a prize. And in a way it is. A diagnosis is a certificate of authenticity; it offers recognition. And, not unimportantly, there are practical advantages: an officially recognised condition means your insurer will cover your treatment and your employer will give you leave to recover. Without the label, neither will be forthcoming.

To cut a long story short, the DSM told me I was ill.

As I hop off the bus in Driebergen, it starts to rain. I try not to see it as a sign. With a hint of reluctance, or perhaps it's more nervous anticipation at facing a packed programme of anxiety-themed activities, I walk to the convention centre that Marina's foundation has hired for the day. She penned her last foreword to *The Phobia Vizier* in 1995. In the preceding decade, her absences had become more frequent. In 1986, she slipped on the pavement and broke her arm. In 1988, she fell down the stairs and bruised a few ribs. In October 1989, another foreword went unwritten when she was hospitalised with severe cardiac problems. A second operation followed in 1990. Precursors of the end became harder to ignore. She feared death, which had been a constant presence during her war years. Over thirty years after the panic attack that had defined the rest of her life, she wrote her final foreword. A contemplative Christmas message, the kind her husband liked to write, about Job and his troubles. "For me, the best comforters are those who can endure sorrow, who are not deterred by your inconsolability, those brave enough to stay with you in the dark." From my own experience, I would like to add that they are not only the best comforters, but also the best friends, family members and lovers. Marina de Wolf-Ferdinandusse died in April 1997.

I arrive at the convention centre to find a group of members raising the foundation's faded flag. A donkey is stationed beside the flagpole. Stroking him is supposed to generate good vibes and ward off the bad. I give it a go; his nose is damp, his eyes doleful. I find it hard not to see animals as people in animal costumes. The person in this costume badly wants to go home. Under other circumstances, I would have marked this memorable moment by taking a selfie with the donkey and sending it to D. (who presumably would have had no idea what to make of it). I take a deep breath and tell myself that I am ready to meet Marina's fellow fearties, people who – without her foundation – might still be stumbling in the dark.

\*

The foyer is buzzing. White crockery is stacked beside coffee urns, trays offer a selection of cheese sticks and gingernuts. Lively clusters of participants swap tips on which seminars to attend. A bell rings and we sweep into the main hall.

The story of the organisation behind the conference – the Anxiety, Compulsion and Phobia Foundation – is not an isolated one. In the UK, the US, Germany, France and other Western countries, foundations focused on fear have undergone a similar evolution. They began with a bunch of sensitive, war-traumatised people in search of ways to handle their fears. This explains the importance they attach to phobias, which are more commonly linked to trauma than to general anxiety. They soon found that problematic anxiety was far more widespread than they had initially thought. Anxiety sufferers sought each other out, forming groups and associations which grew in number. Meanwhile, psychiatry evolved as a profession. The anxiety disorder became commonplace. For every hundred Dutch people who had an anxiety disorder in 1992, there were four hundred and fifty in 2010, according to Maastricht University's Research Network on Family Medicine. Worldwide, estimates by the World Health Organization point to a 15 per cent rise in the number of people with anxiety disorders over the past decade. As already mentioned, such figures may not be entirely accurate but they are the only quantitative guide we have.

As soon as we are seated, a junior minister from the Department of Health takes the floor. Having confessed to a phobia of dams and low-flying zeppelins, he declares the conference open. Pointing at the cameras recording the proceedings, he extends a special welcome to those who are too frightened to leave their homes and are watching from their couch, hoping for that one insight that might make their lives a little easier. For a moment, I fantasise that D. is tuning in and has spotted me here in the second row, notepad on my knees.

Listening to the minister's opening spiel, I have no idea that in a matter of months I will be asked to comment on the rough cut of a TV ad conceived by the Department of Health as part of a new public information campaign about anxiety and phobias. It starts with a series of people waking up and getting dressed. They each put on a black T-shirt with a different label: emetophobic, aviophobic, sociophobic. Then they look into the lens and say a few words about what makes them anxious: vomiting, flying, meeting people. The screen goes black and the campaign slogan swims into view: *you don't have to hide the fear you hold inside.* It is a message I support, in part at least. Talking is almost always better than not talking. Fears fester when consigned to silence. They grow and become harder to handle. At the same time, it occurs to me that using these DSM-approved Latin terms might make people seem more ill than they possibly are: why can't the man in the sociophobic T-shirt just tell us he's shy? Does it help him to think of himself as a medical case? Does it increase his chances of getting better, of participating fully in society once again? In some cases, aren't we simply being made to feel ill? Professor of the Philosophy and History of Science Trudy Dehue draws a parallel with how we classify the animal kingdom. "The difference between domestic animals and livestock raised for slaughter may be arbitrary – for sacred cows, you only need to go to India – but it pretty much determines their fate." Whether Marina's fearties are being domesticated or led to slaughter is a distinction I will leave it to others to make. But it's worth noting that they are becoming increasingly rare in the wild.

Once the minister has done his bit, a twitchy red-haired comic announces the schedule for the day. A few last-minute adjustments have compromised the accuracy of our programmes. "But no need to panic," the comic says. "There's a shitload of oxazepam in the basement." A murmur from the audience. "Seriously," he says with admirable enthusiasm, "we're going to be alright."

I have signed up for a series of speed dates designed to shed an intimate and confrontational light on the phenomenon of anxiety. In a small room with a low, tiled ceiling and a moribund ficus in the corner, I meet Anita (47) and Elisa (21). Mother and daughter have long, blond hair and friendly features that seem to have been sketched using the same template. Anita's story illustrates how deeply intertwined nature and nurture often are. For years, she was so afraid of passing her crippling fears on to the next generation that she didn't want to have children. On discovering she was pregnant, she resolved there and then to keep her fears from her unborn child. When Elisa was born, Anita suffered from postpartum depression, which slowly developed into a state of semi-permanent anxiety. She stuck to her resolution but the strategy backfired. Growing up in a household where fears and anxiety were never discussed, Elisa – who was beginning to develop anxieties of her own – had no-one to turn to. In time, she developed a debilitating fear of vomiting. Anita's fear of passing on her fears to her daughter ultimately became a self-fulfilling prophecy.

We switch tables and Thea (45) sits down opposite me. She suffers from a compulsive disorder. In faltering sentences, almost paralysed by shame, she tells me about her constant fear of hurting someone. Driving along, she feels a small bump in the road and is convinced that she has run someone over. But when she turns the car around, she drives over another pothole and is more sure than ever that now she really has run someone over. The simplest trip can take hours. When she comes home her husband sometimes asks, "Did it happen again?" All Thea can do is nod.

Corinne (39) suffers from agoraphobia. She was working for a multinational when her body began to seize up with cramp. The company doctors thought it was a burnout, but the problem went deeper. Corinne's world steadily shrank; she spoke to fewer and fewer people. Her benefit entitlement is nearing its end and stress is mounting. Without that money coming in, she will be unable to support herself, and she is afraid that starting a new job will be too much for her.

I speak to Anne, Hans, Desirée, Manon and many others. Here they are, those frightened children Marina heard about in the 1980s, the next generation of fearties. A speed date works both ways, of course, and some of my dates ask me about my situation. I stammer the vaguest of replies. I wouldn't know where to start or where to end. More to the point, I have the feeling that if I mention D., I will break beyond repair.

My head is pounding from all these glimpses into lives marked by fear. Lives that still play out within the bounds of what we think of as normal. These are people dealing with their anxieties within society's mainstream, with the help of family, a sound relationship, the care of a doctor. Their fears have not spiralled into psychoses or acts of desperation. They have not fallen through the cracks, they are not a danger to themselves or others. They are here, not in a clinic, an institution or a wooden box. We exchange details and I ask if I can contact them at a later date to ask them some more questions. Their answer is yes. Whether they know it or not, their input is as important to this account as mine. My story is a variation on theirs, their stories are versions of my own.

The afternoon comes to an end and, heading for the cloakroom, I run into the stand-up who was on stage earlier. Pepijn is his name. He makes an immediate impression on me with his open-heartedness backed up by expertise. He talks about combining, upping and reducing dosages, about the stress hormone cortisol, about cycles and swings in the course of a day (most people with heightened anxiety find mornings toughest because our cortisol levels peak before we wake; an evolutionary mechanism to help us start the day alert). We say a hurried goodbye and I make a last-minute dash for my train.

Outside it's raining again, perhaps it never stopped. The donkey has long since been led away. Either that or he made a bid for freedom. On the train, my phone beeps. It's a friend request from Pepijn.

# 9

## *Pepijn's Pills*

Having seen, heard and taken on board so many anguished lives at the conference, I let my world shrink again in the days that follow. I breathe in, I breathe out. The curve of my body is starting to leave an indentation in the mattress as I develop an intimate connection with certain positions; foetal remains a favourite. The loneliness of living without D., alleviated at times by my journey into anxiety, finds expression in new ways. Cold baked beans spooned straight from the can. A dried-up plant that is suddenly waterlogged. The crumpled remains of a clumsily rolled joint (anxiety's not great for your fine motor skills) on the corner of the dining-room table. And then, on a Tuesday evening veiled in mist and rain, Pepijn calls for the first time and insists we have coffee.

Pepijn was born in 1985. There are two ways to tell his story: as tragedy or bitter comedy.

A genuine tragedy begins with a death, and Pepijn's is no different. In this case, the death of his father. Patricius – Patty to everyone who knew him – was an agriculturalist who specialised in plant development. He suffered from insomnia and Crohn's disease, and probably had an anxiety disorder. In 2014 he was diagnosed with Merkel cell carcinoma, a rare and aggressive form of skin cancer. The end came quickly. Not long before, seeing what anxiety was doing to his son, he sighed to Pepijn, "It's you I worry about more than anything. I'm afraid fear will be the death of you."

Four years earlier, Pepijn's GP had diagnosed him with generalised anxiety disorder, a permanently elevated level of anxiety that can shoot up at the slightest trigger. Pepijn had gone to see his doctor about the panic that overcame him on discovering that the top-floor apartment he had just purchased was far too hot. Under that flat roof, which absorbed heat and caused it to linger, he was afraid he might never sleep again. The resulting stress stopped him falling asleep. Exhaustion led to panic. Fear of insomnia became a self-fulfilling prophecy.

The diagnosis came as a relief to Pepijn, as disparate elements from his life story clicked into place. His childhood fear of the way the other boys looked at him when he played in the sandbox. His anxiety as an adolescent when it turned out that his body was not producing growth hormones. The fears he experienced as a young man when he enrolled at drama school in Amsterdam and lived on his own for the first time: the silence of his student lodgings, the competitiveness between students, the loneliness. Each episode of worry and anxiety was given a place in the clear narrative offered by a single diagnosis: he was suffering from a disorder. At the age of twenty-five, Pepijn began taking the antidepressant citalopram to ease his general anxiety, which it did.

The opening scene of the bitter comedy might be the family Christmas when Pepijn's nieces and nephews couldn't stop singing his ex-girlfriend's hit song. Since their break-up, she had reinvented herself as a success. Once she had been the one who looked up to him. He had been the man with the plan, the one who knew how life worked.

They met at a summer theatre festival. An evening of culture in circus tents: it was the last thing Pepijn needed so soon after the death of Patty, the domineering father who cast such a long shadow. Yet there he was talking to this girl and instead of feeling maudlin or lonely, a world of hope opened up for him. With her chunky gold chain and her penchant for football shirts, B. made an indelible impression. Before long, it seemed predestined that their paths should cross on this of all nights, now that his father was no longer looking over his shoulder. After dating for six months, they moved in together and soon they were building a stable home life. Together they handled whatever chance threw at them, talking, laughing, expressing their faith in each other. Pepijn felt firmer ground beneath his feet, less at risk of being knocked sideways. Snuggled up beside his lover, he slept like a baby, her head resting in the cup of his hand. In this new calm, he found the focus and the patience to build an intricate scale model of a Saturn 5 rocket; it took him over a year to turn a mound of jagged plastic pieces into a space-age sculpture that stood proudly next to his computer. Feeling completely secure in this domestic idyll, he started cutting down on his citalopram. A drug-free life was the ideal, after all. Standing on your own two feet. Things were going so well.

Until one day Pepijn noticed a strange whistling whenever he breathed in through his nose. Had it always been there and he was only noticing it now, or had something changed?

'Something's changed, hasn't it?' he asked B. 'This could be really bad. Christ, what could it be?'

B. advised him to see a doctor. This time, the diagnosis was that Pepijn, a habitual nose-picker as a child, had a hole in his septum. Pepijn panicked. He was sure the noise would stop him sleeping. And without sleep, he might lose control or go completely mad. To operate or not to operate? What if something went wrong at the hospital?

Meanwhile, his conversations with B. became strained. He asked for reassurance, she did not respond. No matter, they were made for each together, Pepijn had no doubts on that score.

Until one night B. sighed and told Pepijn that the security he craved simply wasn't what she needed. A bolt from the blue. They stood there for a long time, face to face, and when enough time had passed, they knew it was over. As his breathing quickened, he looked around at the apartment – the home – that would soon be dismantled. His eyes came to rest on the model of Saturn 5. One well-aimed swing and it was back to being a mess of jagged plastic pieces on the floor. "See how easy it is?" he screamed. "To break something beautiful."

Comedy and tragedy converged. A convergence that marked the beginning of a long road that took him to therapists, psychiatrists and, more often than not, to drug stores, pharmacies and assorted dispensers of pills.

Before we step into the psychopharmaceutical vortex for a closer look at the story of Pepijn and his pills, it's worth realising that there are no separate drugs for anxiety and panic disorders. At most, there are anxiety inhibitors for acute panic, and these only work for a short time. For the majority of mental health issues, including anxiety and panic disorders, people are prescribed anti-depressants.

As we know, the first drug Pepijn took was citalopram, an antidepressant often prescribed to people struggling with over-whelming anxiety. Citalopram is a selective serotonin reuptake inhibitor (SSRI), a category of drugs that slow the rate at which the neurotransmitter serotonin is reabsorbed by the body. This lengthens the amount of time it remains active in the brain. (A neurotransmitter is a chemical that transmits impulses between nerve cells, between nerve cells and muscle cells, or between nerve cells and gland cells.) SSRIs accounted for more than half of the over one million antidepressants prescribed in the Netherlands in 2017. Historically, SSRIs (sometimes jokingly called "happy pills") represent the fourth global wave of chemical anti-anxiety medications that reached our shores between the 1940s and the 1970s. Each wave began in the United States and the rest of the West caught the swell. Before these drugs were widely available, people with anxiety often self-medicated with alcohol, marijuana or opium, usually highly diluted and appealingly packaged as a pseudoscientific elixir.

The first wave, in the 1940s, involved barbiturates and meprobamate. Barbiturates are derivatives of barbituric acid, a substance with strong anaesthetic effects on the central nervous system. The first barbiturate was produced in 1864 by a German chemist who combined condensed urea from animal secretions with diethyl malonate derived from malic acid. This compound remained on the shelf until 1903, when researchers at the pharmaceutical company Bayer administered it to dogs and discovered that it put them to sleep in no time. Months later, it was being marketed to humans. This had its drawbacks: barbiturates are highly addictive, shut down entire sections of your mental life, and can all too easily result in a coma or even sudden death, as in the case of Marilyn Monroe. In 1951, *The New York Times* described barbiturates as "more of a menace to society than heroin or morphine". Meprobamate (which belongs to a category of organic compounds called carbamates) is also a sedative, with roughly the same side effects as a barbiturate.

The second wave arrived in the 1950s, following a number of scientific breakthroughs relating to the influence of neurotransmitters on our state of mind. In 1954, Marthe Vogt, a German neuroscientist working in the UK, discovered the role that norepinephrine (also known as noradrenaline) plays as a neurotransmitter in the neurons of the brain. Later that year, during a series of famous experiments, her colleague John Gaddum discovered that LSD lowered the concentration of serotonin in his blood. Since he invariably felt miserable after such an experiment, he concluded that serotonin must have a considerable influence on his mood. In 1955, experiments on rabbits showed that decreased serotonin levels in the blood resulted in lethargic behaviour that was popularly characterised as "depressive": with this, the link between neurochemistry and behaviour entered the public consciousness for the first time.

In 1957, pharmaceutical company Hoffmann-La Roche marketed iproniazid, under the trade name Marsilid, one of the world's first antidepressants. This breakthrough came after TB patients at a New Jersey hospital were given a course of iproniazid in 1952 and wound up dancing down the hallways. Marsilid turned out to have no real effect on TB, and the focus shifted towards using the drug to treat people with depression. The 1950s also saw the first tricyclic antidepressants or TCAs coming onto the market, so called because their chemical structure consists of three rings of atoms. These were found to be beneficial in combating anxiety symptoms by inhibiting the reuptake of serotonin and norepinephrine. TCAs, which are still widely prescribed, can usually be identified by the suffix *ine* (e.g. clomipramine, mirtazapine). In September 1959, *The New York Times* published an article about Marsilid and the first tricyclic drugs, describing them as "antidepressants" – a brand-new term at the time.

The third wave gathered momentum in the 1960s, as the US federal government began providing major financial support to pharmaceutical companies to conduct large-scale studies on the influence of neurotransmitters on mental disorders. In 1963, British psychiatrist Alec Coppen put forward the idea that Marsilid and related drugs increased serotonin levels in the brain. This idea was adopted by the medical profession and with each new adherent, the thinking became less nuanced and the claims bolder. It seemed to capture the spirit of the age and coincided neatly with the aforementioned flow of government funding. The idea, the validity of which has never been proved or even plausibly demonstrated, became an article of faith. Another result of such state-sponsored studies was the emergence of benzodiazepines, a class of drugs whose core chemical structure consists of the fusion of benzene and diazepine. Benzodiazepines, which bolster the effect of the neurotransmitter gamma-aminobutyric acid, had significantly fewer harmful side effects than their predecessors and are still prescribed, especially for short-term use. The best-known examples are tranquilisers such as Valium and virtually all "the pams", as they are sometimes affectionately called. One is oxazepam, the drug Pepijn joked about at the conference where we met.

The 1970s brought the fourth (and to date final) wave of pharmacological breakthroughs in the field of anti-anxiety medication: the advent of the SSRI. The effectiveness of SSRIs centres on the neurotransmitter serotonin, which boosts everything from mood and memory to emotions, sexual activeness and appetite. Though no-one seems to know exactly how it works, serotonin is often associated with feelings of self-esteem and recognition. "But in any case," French writer Michel Houellebecq notes in his novel *Serotonin*, "it is essentially produced within the intestine and it has been found to exist in a great variety of living creatures, including amoebas. What feeling of self-esteem could exist among amoebas? I have gradually reached the conclusion that medical art remains confused and imprecise about these matters . . ." There have been no major pharmacological developments in this field since the 1970s and SSRIs have gradually come to dominate the market in antidepressants. Antibiotics aside, they are thought to be the best-selling drugs in the history of the world.

What should we make of this chemical history in which coincidences, ambiguities and the desire to turn a profit play such a leading role? Today, psychiatrists routinely sketch a fairly straightforward scenario for their patients: you are suffering from a chemical imbalance of the brain and there are drugs that can remedy the problem. As for the exact nature of that imbalance, or what constitutes a chemically balanced brain in the first place, no-one actually knows. To say nothing of the role that antidepressants play in redressing the balance. Then there is the brain's flexibility to consider. It changes constantly, reinforcing the synapses (connections between neurons) we need regularly and allowing less relevant connections to fade away. A brain scan is a snapshot, comparable to a frame on a roll of film. The frame provides us with some information but offers only a limited basis for drawing conclusions, especially in the long term. Ronald Pies, former editor of the magazine *Psychiatric Times*, describes the term chemical imbalance as "a kind of bumper-sticker term that saves time". These time savings are clearly a benefit to psychiatrists and pharmaceutical companies. For patients, the picture is more complex.

Back to Pepijn. Saturn 5 lay in pieces on the floor and B. disappeared from his life.

After her departure, Pepijn lost all sense of purpose. Dazed, he paced from room to room or roamed the streets of his neighbourhood. When he picked up a newspaper, he found no logic in what he read. The world had become incomprehensible, a shift so sudden that he could no longer recall what comprehension felt like or how being alone worked. B.'s departure had punched holes in his home and shrouded even his own belongings in a cold light. He was a stranger to himself. News of her life without him trickled through: photos of parties, premieres, successes, no sign of regrets. Was he the only one mourning what they had lost, giving it the send-off it deserved? Safety was nowhere to be found and Pepijn began calling friend after friend, constantly seeking reassurance. His dying father's words about succumbing to fear were feeling more ominous by the day.

He was in over his head, jolting awake every morning, sick with panic. It was time to start taking his pills again. But citalopram, the drug that had once worked so well for him, no longer had an effect; his body seemed to have become resistant. He and his psychiatrist had to find an alternative, a search that launched Pepijn into a game of pharmaceutical pinball that continues to this day. The grand pinball prize, the ultimate high score, being the perfect drug for him.

Unfortunately, the perfect drug is almost always an illusion. No two bodies react the same to any given medicine and the process is invariably one of trial and error: gauging the initial effect and then increasing or reducing the dosage. The next drug Pepijn was prescribed was oxazepam, in combination with venlafaxine, a serotonin-norepinephrine reuptake inhibitor or SNRI. This class of drugs ensures that, in addition to serotonin, the neurotransmitter norepinephrine remains active longer. (Norepinephrine is similar to adrenaline and has a mood-enhancing effect.) Pepijn stuck with this regime for four months, though the venlafaxine gave him such severe stomach aches that he was unable to walk upright.

Time for a new drug, and Pepijn was prescribed an SSRI called sertraline. The drug didn't work and left a nasty, bitter taste in his mouth. At times it felt like his tongue was on fire. This went on for six weeks, the minimum to determine whether or not sertraline was having the desired effect.

On to another candidate: fluvoxamine, another SSRI. This did nothing at all to lift his spirits but fogged his mind and blurred his vision to the extent that he was scared to ride his bike. Another six-week stint.

Next up was mirtazapine, a tetracyclic antidepressant, which worked but came with a host of unpleasant side effects. Pepijn gained eight pounds in three weeks. His memory became patchy, his mouth was always dry, and nothing he experienced seemed to stick. If something startled him – an unexpected noise was enough – it felt like an electric shock.

Six weeks later it was the turn of escitalopram, a relatively new drug (2011) with strong similarities to citalopram (1989). Other than a difference in the three-dimensional orientation of the active isomers (left handed or right handed), it was the price that set it apart: escitalopram was the most expensive SSRI on the market at the time. Unfortunately, the drug did very little for Pepijn; he remained just as anxious and worried. After three months, it was time for a change.

He decided to add nortriptyline, another tricyclic antidepressant, to unsettling effect. Pepijn was thrown into a confused, intensely nervous and highly emotional state that drove him to the brink of madness. He felt a constant urge to escape, without knowing what from. He stuck it out for two weeks.

A month on agomelatine followed, a drug similar to the sleep hormone melatonin, but this made Pepijn feel queasy all the time. He walked around with his head spinning, and his sleep was fitful at best.

An exhaustive account, designed to wear you down just a little and give you some idea of what this must have been like for Pepijn, to say nothing of the impact on his brain, that finely tuned system of some 450,000 kilometres of wiring, with between five and ten thousand trillion interconnections (more than the estimated number of stars in the observable universe).

At the end of all this, Pepijn started on duloxetine, another SNRI. Months later, he is still popping the pills. They work, to some extent at least, and the side effects are manageable. That said, for the first two months he had no libido. Zilch. He would go out on a date, end up in the sack with the woman of his dreams only to feel no physical response whatsoever. It was as if his cock had bailed out on him. For a while now, it's been better. For a while now, it's not been so bad.

My phone rings. It's Pepijn. There are days when his are the only calls I pick up. There are days when he's the only one who calls.

Let's head back to the 1990s, when Pepijn was still a kid. A time that came to be known as The Age of the Brain. Our destination is the Jelgersma Clinic: a beautiful art nouveau building in a Dutch woodland setting which, at the start of last century, opened its doors to members of the middle classes who were suffering with their nerves. In 1995, the clinic became the focus of a documentary series featuring an up-and-coming professor who was about to transform the field of psychiatry. René Kahn, an affiliate of Utrecht University, was seen as a champion of "biological psychiatry", a new, more business-like take on the profession. As its name suggests, biological psychiatry is founded on the notion that, since our behaviour is anchored in the brain, changes to the brain can bring about changes in behaviour. These changes could be effected by a long-term intervention in the shape of psychotherapy and behavioural therapy sessions, but also most definitely by drugs. During his specialist training in the early 1980s, Kahn had studied a number of articles from the US and the UK about the effectiveness of clomipramine, better known by its brand name Anafranil. This was an eye-opener: the first accounts he had read of a drug that appeared to be successful in treating what were then called neurotic disorders. Kahn's interest was piqued, not so much by anxiety as a phenomenon, but by the prospect of innovation and solutions.

When I meet René Kahn, he is on a brief working visit to a Utrecht hospital, far from his day job as a professor at New York's prestigious Mount Sinai Hospital. I ask him why he has never really wanted to fathom the nature of anxiety. His answer is characteristically blunt: "Why would I? I'm a doctor, not a philosopher."

Having qualified as a doctor, Kahn left for New York, where the discipline of psychiatry had pretty much turned its back on psychoanalytic discourse. The future was digital. All that chat between doctor and patient was old hat; the focus now was on obtaining facts and generating data, taking an evidence-based, demonstrably scientific approach. Kahn specialised in pharmacological research that used digital scanning and imaging technology to create 3D models that could show the loci of brain activity. Kahn was convinced that this biological route was the way to go and, when he was lured back to work in the Netherlands, he wasted no time asserting those convictions in his homeland.

Of course, this new approach didn't materialise out of nowhere; it was a sea change rather than a lightning strike. In the early 1980s, the tide was already turning, as reflected by the opinions expressed in Marina de Wolf-Ferdinandusse's foundation and its magazine *The Phobia Vizier*. At the very start of the decade, Marina appeared on a TV current affairs show to talk about "the panic pill", a new drug that had been shown to alleviate panic attacks. Her foundation was in close contact with universities in Groningen and

Utrecht, monitoring the effects of this antidepressant on members who had signed up for clinical trials. Studies like these prompted an angry response from some of Marina's fearties, indignant at being "pressganged" into becoming test subjects. But Marina was convinced of the value of the panic pill. One contribution to a 1992 edition of the magazine backs her to the hilt: a member called Minou writes that the scientist who discovered Fevarin (a precursor to fluvoxamine, one of the drugs prescribed to Pepijn twenty years later) should have a statue erected in his honour. "And while we're at it, my deepest gratitude to whoever is pulling the strings up there." The pill as a godsend. In 1994, the brand name Prozac appeared for the first time in the pages of *The Phobia Vizier*.

In 1995, it was lights, camera, action for the documentary crew at the Jelgersma Clinic. "If it's matters of the soul you're after, you are talking to the wrong man," René Kahn told the interviewer with the unshakeable assurance of an iconoclast and medical messiah rolled into one. Coolly, he assured viewers that his combination of brain scans and pharmaceuticals would rid 80 to 90 per cent of those under his care of their depressive symptoms.

"Eighty to ninety per cent?" the interviewer asked incredulously.

"Yes," Kahn replied.

"But that would take years, surely?"

"No-o," Kahn replied, dragging out the vowel as if the question had been asked for the umpteenth time by one of his more obtuse students. "Not years. If the patient responds to treatment immediately, it will take three months." Kahn estimated that around 60 per cent of patients would show an immediate response. "The point is that psychiatry, like the rest of the medical world, is now becoming scientific and measurable. In the past, it was too much of an art, a philosophy."

Kahn's promise resonated with the general public. He appealed to our desire for clarity, and the combination of his words and his attitude fuelled our hope for tangible results that were also affordable. Kahn's calm insistence tilted our perspective. Suddenly, the vague psychologising of the past felt foolishly old-fashioned. Chat was old hat; the psyche had been taken out of psychiatry.

In the intervening period, drugs have become the most common solution to mental health problems. "The truth is that patients often have very little patience," Damiaan Denys, President of the Dutch Association for Psychiatry explains. "And we psychiatrists have very little time. Generally speaking, that makes it both statistically and socially more desirable to start with medication, and then to see if there's a need for additional therapies." While this sounds plausible enough, I can't help wondering whether it might run counter to one of the guiding principles of medicine: *primum non nocere*. Loosely translated, if you can't heal someone, at least make every effort not to harm them.

Psychopharmaceuticals, drugs once developed to treat truly severe cases – people who could not function without them and were in danger of going under – are now being taken by masses of patients, including some who could actually do without them. This certainly applies to anxiety. And since anxiety can never be solved (in the sense that new fears and worries will always emerge), from a psychopharmaceutical perspective it represents an inexhaustible source of income. Revenues can be secured with a smart patenting policy. Patents on drugs expire after a number of years, but companies can have them extended by making minimal changes to a drug's make-up or tweaking an irrelevant aspect of the manufacturing process. This perfectly legal manipulation is called "evergreening": repatenting a particular medicine makes sure that it remains profitable. The full extent of this practice was only studied for the first time recently, by law professor Robin Feldman. She succeeded in obtaining a decade's worth of data from the US Food and Drug Administration (FDA) and went through it with a fine-toothed comb. Her conclusion: 78 per cent of the drugs that had been patented as new were actually old. The purpose of evergreening, which Feldman's research shows is becoming increasingly common, could not be clearer: as long as a drug is patented, the manufacturer effectively holds a monopoly on its production and the price can be kept artificially high.

A particularly flagrant example of how to exploit such a monopoly concerns the drug Syprine, which is taken to lower copper levels in the blood. A standard dose of Syprine cost 650 US dollars in 2010. After a five-year period during which parent company Valeant drove up the price, Syprine cost more than 21,000 US dollars. Valeant could afford to do so because no competitor was in a position to offer an alternative. And the patient was left to foot the bill.

What made Kahn and his cohorts so sure of their approach? Was their self-confidence justified, or was it hubris? Plenty of positive studies on the effects of antidepressants were available at the time. And those studies, a number of which Kahn had read, were reliable, weren't they?

Former GP and renowned epidemiologist Dick Bijl begs to differ. "Many of those studies have shortcomings. Rather a lot of shortcomings, in fact." Bijl, President of the International Society of Drug Bulletins, is one of a rare breed: an independent medical professional who has dedicated himself to fathoming the ins and outs of drug research. Over the last twenty-two years, he has read and commented on some thirty thousand publications. In his view, many such studies are rush jobs (a trial often runs for less than twelve weeks) that are poorly conducted. On top of this, there is the phenomenon of "publication bias": for decades, pharmaceutical companies have released only those studies with positive results, even though some of the drugs patients like Pepijn are still taking have generated far more negative than positive findings. Of all the drug studies conducted by pharmaceutical companies, up to 40 per cent have never been released at all, while the remaining 60 per cent are subject to highly selective publication practices. In an interview for Dutch television, psychiatrist Bram Bakker said, "For years, people who stopped taking the medication early on because it didn't work or led to unpleasant side effects were not included in the study." Today, a pharmaceutical company only has to come up with two positive studies to have a drug approved. It is therefore conceivable that a drug that has had no effect in seventy studies and a positive effect in two can find its way to market.

The history of the world's most famous antidepressant, Prozac, is a case in point. During the trial period, the drug was dispensed to 245 patients. But the pharmaceutical company only released the results of twenty-seven patients, all of whom had responded positively to the drug. The rest of the results have always been kept out of the public domain. And once a drug is on the market, it is very rare for additional research to be done.

"I prefer to speak in terms of medicines rather than cures," Dick Bijl says. "The truth is that most drugs don't cure anything at all." As he sees it, we are obsessed with statistics, which are open to manipulation, and fail to take a sufficient interest in how those statistics relate to the real world. "An effect can be statistically significant and still make no difference to the patient." He is referring to the Hamilton Depression Scale, which assigns a score to a person's state of mind based on a questionnaire. The scores run from 0 to 52: the higher your score, the more severe your condition. People with depression tend to score around 20. "To know whether or not an antidepressant works, you need to compare it to a fake pill, a placebo. On average, an antidepressant lowers the score from 20 to 12."

Time to break out the Prozac? Not quite.

"A placebo lowers the score to 13: a one-point difference from the real drug. Include enough people in your study and you can call that one point significant. But what does that mean? Not a great deal."

Professor Irving Kirsch of Harvard Medical School, initially a strong proponent of antidepressants, also concluded on the basis of a 1998 study of the placebo effect in antidepressants that subjects given these drugs fared only marginally better than those given placebos. His extensive research showed that 25 per cent of the effect of antidepressants could be ascribed to natural recovery, 50 per cent to patient expectations about the effectiveness of antidepressants, and only 25 per cent to the chemical effect of the drug itself. At this point, it's important to note that in 25 per cent of cases these substances *were* shown to be effective. There are plenty of people who can tell you how these drugs have changed their lives for the better.

However many times Irving revisited and recalculated the results, he could not escape the conclusion to which they led: it was time to topple the edifice he had helped build with dozens of positive articles about the effectiveness of antidepressants. "One thing I do pride myself on," he later told British journalist Johann Hari, "is looking at the data, and allowing my mind to be changed when the data's different than I expected." Following an additional study in 2008, Kirsch found that the pills work primarily in patients with a very severe depressive disorder. The conclusions he reached in these leading studies have never been undermined.

Why do these medicines so often fail to do what is expected of them? In addition to our collective ignorance of exactly how SSRIs work – as expressed in Houellebecq's amoeba quote – leading American neuroscientist Joseph LeDoux cites another fundamental reason for their shortcomings: antidepressants essentially dampen our responses without removing our anxiety. To explain this, I have to go back to the difference between the fear reflex we share with other animals (whereby the amygdala sends the body into fight/ flight/freeze mode) and our distinctly human experience of fear, with its strong links to language, imagination and self-awareness (all facilitated by the prefrontal cortex). Keep that difference in mind.

SSRIs are tested in animal experiments, usually by exposing mice to threatening situations. It works something like this: if the endangered mice appear less timid after being administered a certain antidepressant and if their cortisol levels drop, the drug is assumed to be working. This observation then forms the basis for an assumption which appears logical but is actually wide of the mark: we assume that a drug that is successful in mice will have the same effect in humans, because we also have an amygdala. But in reaching this conclusion we bypass the subjective side of fear and the role played by the human prefrontal cortex.

How we perceive and experience a threat – the aspects of fear that revolve around self-awareness and imagination – are not part of the equation when SSRIs are tested. The same is true of feelings of insecurity and anxiety in relation to perceived threats that are not concrete. These are mainly processed not by the amygdala but by the bed nucleus of the stria terminalis (BNST), a kind of gateway to the amygdala. Because the BNST is far less developed in laboratory animals than it is in humans, we can conclude that animal experiments have little to contribute to our understanding and treatment of people who simply have an anxious disposition.

Ever since the 1950s, animal experiments with all their limitations have been the primary method of testing anti-anxiety medications, and so for decades we have been trying to treat anxiety in humans with agents that appear to tackle fear in animals. "It's led to the development of medications that don't really work," LeDoux says. "They are targeted to work on these underlying systems in rats and in mice but that's not where we are experiencing our anxiety." While pointing out that the drugs available can help people by "turning down the volume" on their responses, he explains that this is a crude and indiscriminate intervention: the active chemicals not only affect the parts of the brain that produce anxiety hormones, but also the parts that coordinate other vital processes such as memory and attention.

My own feelings about antidepressants are mixed. I write this having just swallowed my little white oval for the day, the familiar bitter taste followed by the burning chemical trail down my throat. I still remember the first meds I was prescribed. Three pills to be taken daily: an antidepressant (SSRI), an anxiety inhibitor and a sleeping pill (tricyclic). During those first days on pharmaceuticals, it was as if all my senses were being recalibrated: my ears were ringing, my eyesight deteriorated, my stomach ached and I felt incredibly tired. But it wasn't all bad: I had my first good night's sleep in years.

Very occasionally, if she had trouble sleeping, D. would take one of my pills. Once, in the middle of the night, I heard rustling and looked up to see her shuffling out of the bedroom. I found her in my study, her sweet body illuminated by a street lamp outside; she slept naked, something I could never bring myself to do. She opened a drawer, found the box of pills. Her head tipped back as she swallowed. I cherished the acceptance I saw in those moments. In taking my medicine, it felt like she was taking my side.

Let me be clear: in severe cases, antidepressants can have a huge impact. The right pill at the right time can be the difference between life and death. They have helped me too. At crucial moments, they smoothed over part of my sensitivity, my tendency to fear. My anxiety level would go down and my ability to think and function improved. But dealing with the many side effects can be hard and, like most people who take prescription drugs long term, I regularly find myself asking serious questions that eat away at my confidence. Can I still make it on my own? What am I worth without the pills? Am I still myself, now that my emotions are regulated by chemicals? Thoughts that start as pinpricks but soon gain traction as the daily dose and the two cups of coffee to wash away the taste become a ritual that spans months and then years. And I am not alone in these thoughts.

\*

When we arrange to meet, Pepijn invariably turns up late with the woe-begotten expression of someone who has come straight from a catastrophic job interview. He appears skittish, as if constantly on the lookout for ways to keep his fears at bay. His chronic lack of understanding borders on despair. How can he feel this way?

What's happening to him? Is this normal? Is there any way out? "I can't take it anymore," he sighs. "Can't keep this up. I'm so anxious I can barely walk." One evening, five minutes after we've paid the bill at the local Vietnamese, he asks me what I'm having for dinner. Pepijn is stuck in his own thoughts, his own inner world.

From Pepijn I learn that, roughly speaking, anxious people fall into two groups: clingers and loners. The loners try to find their own solutions, increasingly distancing themselves from others and running the risk of becoming not only loners but lonely into the bargain, a path that ultimately leads to bitterness. The clingers hurl themselves at their loved ones and run the risk of alienating them. I don't need to tell you which camp Pepijn belongs to. I too am a clinger at heart. I know this and try to correct my behaviour. As a result, I can seem remote one minute and throw myself at someone's feet the next, when the staying power to maintain an artificial distance deserts me. So far, there has always been a friend willing to take my call. But I know that if enough people don't pick up, I will end up spilling my guts to the guy at the corner shop. Once, after practically begging my friend Kees to go with me to some party, he replied, "It's not a friend you need, it's a guide dog."

With Pepijn, I sometimes settle for the role of guide dog. He deserves to have days without fear, and one day they will be back. And at times it's a privilege to be in a position to help someone, to say things that matter. Albeit briefly, it feels like I am having an undeniably positive influence on someone's life. All the more reason to remain calm. When he calls, I steer him back towards normality, sentence by sentence, word by word. And sometimes he asks me how I'm doing. I tell him about D. and our conversation in the kitchen, about her sleeping somewhere else now, about how sometimes it's as if the apartment blames me for the quiet that has settled in. And then I stop talking.

One Saturday morning, just as I am sitting down to breakfast and a Batman movie, Pepijn calls again. He sounds almost incoherent, sobbing, gulping for air. He is out on his balcony, staring down, afraid of what might happen next. I ask him if he's planning to do something. He says he isn't. I tell him I'm taking him at his word and trusting him not to do anything stupid. He hums in agreement. I invite him – practically order him – to come over, hoping that a walk in the open air will do him good. Thirty minutes tick past and there's no sign of him. I send him a concerned text message. After another thirty minutes, just as I'm putting on my shoes to go and look for him, he appears at last in all his trembling, red-haired glory. After a rambling conversation about what it's like to live alone in a house made for two, he curls up on my couch and falls asleep. It's four in the afternoon. There he lies, knees tucked beneath his chin, sweater bunched up to reveal a pale crescent of lower back. For a second, I see myself lying there, same couch, same position, after hearing from D. that she won't be coming back. The more I think about it, the less I can tell fear from premonition.

This is how Pepijn lives when life becomes a struggle. He clings to those who are loyal to him: his friends, his sister. A psychiatrist told him to call anytime, so he does. Psychiatrists have helped him on many occasions but, presumably at his express request, they mostly dealt him drugs.

Over the years, Pepijn explains days later, he has tried everything. "Meditation, primal scream therapy, family constellations, hugging, mindfulness, lying on a couch visualising paternal archetypes, walking with a horse to ground myself. But after a while I always wound up thinking: what the hell am I doing?" Pause for thought. "Recently, I've been seeing a coach. He says that, as a child, you experience all kinds of unpleasant things and develop mechanisms to avoid feeling that same pain later. I have to put the things that scare me on islands: worry islands. The side effects of the drugs are one worry island. So, when I catch myself thinking about them, I have to tell myself, 'No, that's a worry island: don't go there.'"

This idea comes from the school of cognitive behavioural

therapy, which treats thoughts as a form of behaviour that needs to be actively steered in a given direction: redirect them often enough and they become less persistent. This approach has its critics, people who object to labelling certain thoughts as wrong and in need of correction. In fact, most studies show that CBT is about as effective as medication when it comes to anxiety disorders, but with less chance of relapse.

Very occasionally, Pepijn tells his "shrink guy" that he wants to stop taking his meds altogether. "My body needs a break from that crap. Anything else is fine: therapy, training, but no more pills." Then his shrink explains that therapy will only have an effect if Pepijn's anxiety level is a little lower, so they end up agreeing to wait and see for a while. Recently, a new drug was added to the mix: Wellbutrin, an antidepressant that slows the absorption of the neurotransmitters norepinephrine and dopamine. Its effects are supposed to be similar to duloxetine – Pepijn's tenth pill – but without the demoralising effect on the libido. At one stage, Pepijn seriously considered having himself admitted to an open facility for a week or two. But his shrink insisted that admission only helps in the severest of cases, when the "case" in question becomes a danger to themselves or to others. Thankfully, Pepijn has never felt the urge to harm anyone, himself included.

Does he regret pumping all those chemicals into his body?

"To be honest, if I'd known what lay ahead, it's hard to imagine I would have started taking the pills," Pepijn admits. "But there's no point thinking like that. It only makes a guy anxious."

It is a bitter but understandable conclusion. René Kahn once promised that antidepressants would free 80 to 90 per cent of patients of their symptoms in a matter of months. We now know better. During our interview in Utrecht, I confront him with the view that the biological approach hasn't really helped us.

"That's a justified criticism," Kahn nods. "Twenty-five years of biological psychiatry has given us all sorts of things. We under- stand far more about the brain. But it has not led to important new treatments for schizophrenia, depression and anxiety disorders. There are three reasons for this. First, the pharmaceutical industry has no real incentive to make such a breakthrough. Economically, it makes more sense for large pharmaceutical companies to tweak an already existing drug and slap the words 'new' and 'improved' on the packaging. That way you generate the revenue without having to fork out for the research. Second, we still don't have the tools to fully understand the brain. And third, having those tools wouldn't necessarily put us in a position to cure depression. Even for diseases with an unambiguous cause observable within the brain, such as Alzheimer's or Huntington's disease, we haven't succeeded in converting our understanding into effective treatment. All told, biological psychiatry has not brought us any major breakthroughs in real terms. And that's a pity."

Has he ever taken this personally? Does he feel that he has failed?

"Oh no," he replies. "That's how science works."

But doesn't he regret making such bold statements?

Again, the answer is no. "If you have a point to make, you have to be one-dimensional about it. People don't want to think too hard, they want black or white. If I had lost myself in nuances and hedged my bets, no-one would have listened. And the point I was making was important. Don't forget that we're talking about a time when people still believed that panic disorder was caused by hyperventilation syndrome. Blowing into a bag and that kind of nonsense. In the years since, I've tried to be more nuanced, but when you take that approach journalists can't get off the phone quickly enough." Hate the game, not the player, is Kahn's message.

Be that as it may, I suspect that Pepijn would have liked to hear more about those nuances before his time as a pinball began. These days, he is working on a model of the International Space Station. One day perhaps, when he's good and ready, he will love someone enough to smash it into tiny pieces.

With over half my journey behind me, I am building a model of my own. One I hope will answer a very complex question that we have touched on already: have people really become more anxious over the years?

Earlier, I looked at how the looping effect can lead to an increase in the prevalence of a condition. But in light of Pepijn's personal history, I realise there must be more to it than that. The fact that the label "anxiety disorder" was so readily adopted in the 1980s and may have been subject to inflation as soon as it was coined, does not rule out the possibility that people have actually become more fearful. The willingness to apply a label does not preclude an increase in the issues that gave rise to the label in the first place. Looking back at my own life, the fears I experienced as a kid, a schoolboy and a student existed long before I had any notion of an anxiety disorder. That said, every century from the seventeenth to the twenty-first has at some point been christened "the age of fear". So what is going on? Marina saw the emergence of a generation of unusually anxious children, a generation to which Pepijn and I belong. Was that an acute observation or was she seeing things?

The figures on officially recognised anxiety disorders offer no satisfying answer to this question. The label is still too new to allow meaningful comparisons. It therefore makes more sense to look at self-reported cases: not anxiety as registered by a doctor, but as reported by sufferers themselves. For this we can look to the United States, and given that the biggest social, economic and cultural changes in post-war American life roughly correspond to those in the rest of the Western world, what we find should be highly relevant to us as well.

It was US psychology professor Jean Twenge who, having heard many accounts of an increase in anxiety, decided to set up a large-scale comparative study in 2000, the first of its kind. The key question: were schoolchildren and students in the United States more anxious in the 1980s than their predecessors had been? Twenge examined over one hundred and seventy relevant studies, covering forty thousand students and twelve thousand schoolchildren between the ages of nine and seventeen, who had reported experiencing excessive anxiety between the 1950s and the year 2000, either to a medical professional or to their school or college. There were a number of criteria: the school or college they attended had to be in the US, the sample had to represent both male and female students, and the pupils/students could not be enrolled in counselling or group therapy.

The results were astounding. Compared to their counterparts in the 1950s, both schoolchildren and students appeared to be increasingly fearful. The increase is linear, but the line gets steeper, especially in the 1970s and 1980s. Student anxiety increased a whole standard deviation between the 1950s and 1990s, about 20 per cent. The graph for schoolchildren follows exactly the same pattern as that for the students. Twenge's shocking conclusion: average schoolchildren in the 1980s were experiencing greater anxiety than child psychiatric patients from a study in the 1950s. No matter how many times she repeated her research and expanded her research group, no matter how many external researchers she brought in to check things over, the results came out the same. Our anxiety levels continued to rise into the 1990s, then stabilised, only to rise again in the second decade of the twenty-first century. (Some philosophers have referred to the period of relative calm between 1989 – the fall of the Berlin Wall, which marked the end of the Cold War – and 2008 – the collapse of Lehman Brothers, which marked the end of the illusion of unending economic prosperity – as the *interanxietas* or interbellum of fear.)

In short, Twenge's figures fit seamlessly with the suspicions of Marina de Wolf-Ferdinandusse, who was no scientist but had a keen sense of what was taking place among her fellow fearties. Which brings me to the question of how to explain this undeniable increase.

# 10

# *From Solidarity to Solitary*
## *(First lesson from the football pitch)*

A square in Amsterdam's old Olympic district. Tall trees sway gently around three football pitches hemmed in by the homes of the well-to-do. I park my bike at a safe distance and stroll in through the dark green gate. This is the club where I played for over half my life, yet entering the grounds always comes with a nervous twist, the result of a painful encounter twenty-five years ago. It was a Wednesday, late summer. Dinner that night would probably have been spaghetti smothered in a jar of carbonara sauce, spiked with extra salt. Black Rucanor bag slung over my shoulder, I arrived for the first training session of the season. Stepping onto the pitch, I saw only unfamiliar faces. Friends who had long since signed up were already being put through their paces elsewhere. Do my best today and I might join them on one of the junior teams. Things got off to a decent enough start and most of what we did was within my capabilities. There was one odd thing: a little guy called Japie would shout over to me every so often and grin broadly. Ladders? Ladas? I couldn't make him out. I eventually plumped for "badass" and took it as a compliment. It was the first session after all. We barely knew each other.

When training was over, I ambled back to my bike, feeling

pretty pleased with myself. Fumbling for my key in the dead zone between the bike rack and the changing rooms, I heard "Ha! Lard Arse!" Japie's unmistakable drawl, followed by howls of laughter. I froze and prayed no-one could see me, racking my brain for a positive or even neutral take on what I had just heard. There wasn't one. Of course Japie knew my name – I knew his, didn't I? He just didn't think a body like mine deserved one. It was months before I dared to show my face again. Ever since, whenever I meet someone new, there is always a fleeting moment when I picture them turning to a friend later and going "So, what did you make of Lard Arse?"

I push the memory aside, as I have done a thousand times before. Today the club is swarming with budding footballers and their parents, juniors and veterans, visitors and home teams. I started here as a schoolboy and played my last match as a thirty-something. I exchange nods with someone I vaguely recognise or who vaguely recognises me, a split-second acknowledgement of the half-forgotten past we share. I climb the stairs to the cafeteria for a view across all three pitches. Why exactly am I here? It's not the most obvious place to ponder one of the trickiest but most important questions on my journey: why have we become more afraid?

To gain a genuine understanding of today's anxious souls (whether or not they have been labelled as such by the DSM), we need to bring together a few fields of study that tend to be viewed separately. The movements that spurred this rise in anxiety have occurred on a grand scale and span a wide range, from philosophy and politics to economics and sociology. These are global developments not immediately apparent in the everyday life of one individual or the events of a single day, processes that affected millions of lives a little at a time until those lives changed for good. This multiplicity makes it tempting to oversimplify, to point to one particular cause of "the anxiety epidemic", as psychiatrists and psychologists in the public arena are wont to do. Dirk De Wachter argues that we have forgotten how to be unhappy. Paul Verhaeghe puts the blame almost entirely on neoliberalism. Damiaan Denys emphasises our obsession with perfectionism. They all have a point and they also make it easy on themselves by focusing on a part of the puzzle while other equally important factors go unmentioned or are even dismissed altogether. I have no appetite for simplifications; we fearties deserve better.

Fortunately for us, many of these global developments can be illustrated on a much smaller scale. And it so happens that one of the settings where they come together is the football club where I spent hundreds of hours of my life.

I leave the cafeteria and head downstairs, past a bulletin board hung with dozens of urgently worded appeals: volunteers are needed to work bar shifts, referee matches, organise tournaments, pump up footballs. Some of these notices are yellowing at the edges. What was it that motivated people to take on these roles in the past? What need did these duties fill that no longer seems to exist?

It has been five years since I called it quits. The veteran team I played for decided to make the move to another club, which gave me a good excuse to announce my retirement. To be honest, I had been looking for one for years. Let's just say that the gap between ability and ambition had been widening at an alarming rate. But the reason for the team's departure is significant: membership was becoming too expensive. Not that anyone was struggling to make the payments, but the combination of a sizeable fee and the obligation to work shifts at the club cafeteria had begun to rankle: six times a year, the team had to delegate players to serve behind the bar. Had the fee been lower, my teammates reasoned, we might have been able to muster the enthusiasm to work those bar shifts, with their soundtrack of hamburgers popping in hot grease and the despondent gurgle of the deep fat fryer. Surely for the amount we were coughing up each month the club could hire people to take care of all that?

We were not alone in our mindset. "The older generation lived for their football club," said Jan Dirk van der Zee of the Dutch Football Association (KNVB) in an interview with national daily *NRC Handelsblad*. "Today's parents are more individualistic. They work long hours, have busy schedules." Van der Zee, the man in charge of the amateur side of the sport, goes on to provide the perfect summation of our team's discontent: people nowadays have gone from being members to consumers.

Football exec Van der Zee shows you don't need to be a philosopher to highlight a crucial shift in society. Perhaps the most famous illustration of this Western phenomenon comes from Harvard-based political scientist Robert Putnam, who studied the declining membership numbers of bowling clubs and the Boy Scouts in the United States. The central image of his bestseller *Bowling Alone* (2000) is that a society once composed of molecules has disintegrated into atoms. From a sense of solidarity, we have gradually withdrawn into solitary existences: every man for himself. The Boy Scouts are dying out, the bowling alleys are deserted, the sports club cafe is understaffed.

What exactly is the difference between a member and a consumer, to stick with Van der Zee's distinction? Consumers look out for their own interests and pay an agreed price for products and services; beyond that, they barely have any responsibilities. But this is an attitude with serious drawbacks. Social cohesion – the connection between institutions, prevailing norms and values, and the members of the group – is dead in the water if people see themselves solely as consumers. A group of consumers amounts to nothing more than a collection of loners.

This gradual historical change, from solidarity to a solitary lifestyle, can be observed at almost every level of society. Demographically speaking, all Western countries have increasingly high divorce rates and fewer births. From a geographical perspective, smaller communities are dying out as younger generations gravitate towards cities, where an increasing proportion of them live alone. In 1950, nine per cent of Americans lived alone; in 2010 that figure was twenty-eight per cent. In 1947, there were three hundred thousand one-person households in the Netherlands; today there are three million.

Shifts like these affect our anxiety levels. You are almost twice as likely to have an anxiety disorder if you live alone than if you cohabit. Recent follow-up research has shown this to be a matter of causation rather than simple correlation. (A correlation shows that two phenomena occur in conjunction, which opens up the possibility of a causal relationship but does not offer proof of one. To speak of causation, there has to be clear evidence that one set of circumstances results from the other.) People who do not have a mental health problem but do feel lonely have a greatly increased chance of developing a serious mood disorder, anxiety disorder or problem with substance abuse within a number of years. You are also almost twice as likely to have an anxiety disorder if you live in a big city, where you encounter more stimuli, experience greater financial and social pressures, and generally lead a more hectic life.

On the religious front: in 2018, Statistics Netherlands reported that, for the first time in history, the number of Dutch people who did not belong to a religious group (51 per cent) outnumbered those who did. In 2012, this had only been the case for 46 per cent of the population. As for politics, the membership of political parties has been in serious decline in almost all Western countries for decades.

Across the board, official figures provide incontrovertible evidence of the dwindling importance of the group and the fading relevance of traditional institutions. This move away from collective endeavour has had many positive effects but has also left a serious dent in our sense of social cohesion. In the Netherlands, the conclusion of a 2008 study on social cohesion, the country's largest to date, pulled no punches: "The Dutch have become more insecure over the years." The respondents thought standards of decency were "plummeting", while values such as solidarity with underprivileged groups, respect for others and tolerance were "being eroded" or "had given way to negative tendencies such as individualism". This, they believed, had led to "selfishness, materialism and aggression".

There is a direct link between social cohesion and how happy people are with the circumstances in which they live: the greater the social cohesion in a neighbourhood, a city or a country, the happier and less anxious people are. By placing more emphasis on our own interests and less on those of the group, we have partly lost our ability to connect with each other. Yet at the same time, our existential need for contact, familiarity and shared values will never disappear: humans are social animals. A more appealing but less common term for social cohesion is "art of association", coined by political scientist Francis Fukuyama. Our mastery of that art has declined over the years, but without association we have nothing to hold on to. And a world that offers nothing to hold on to is a terrifying place.

I wander past the club changing rooms and a familiar dankness drifts towards me: the smell of sweat, dodgy plumbing, wet towels stuffed into sports bags. That used to be my world, I used to smell like that.

It's a grey day. Gulls trace slow circles above the playing fields. On pitch No. 2, a whistle blows and two teams of ten-year-old boys spring into action. The match is scrappy, loss of possession all over the shop. As the nil-nil score line persists and the hunger for a deciding goal intensifies, I start to notice something. Each player seems to think it's up to him to break the deadlock, to push for that ultimate solo. A half-hearted pass leaves the ball stranded in no man's land. The players size each other up: who fancies their chances? A boy in pink football boots and a pristine strip steps up to the mark: snow-white shirt, creaseless shorts, socks pulled up to his knees. One resolute glance at the opponent's goal and he's off. My eyes home in as he starts his run, the rest fade into the background. There's a real beauty in his desire, something we take so much for granted these days that we don't always notice it: the conviction that he is able and entitled to make a difference. It's our acceptance of the individual who wants to set themselves apart, the licence we give a player to see themselves as special, perhaps even unique, at a given moment. How fitting it seems that the boy on the ball should seize this opportunity to prove his exceptionalism, demand the right to fulfil his potential. This right goes to the heart of the belief that facilitated our leap from solidarity to a solitary existence: individualism.

It is hard to say exactly when we began to embrace individualism. The emphasis on individuality has been present to a greater or lesser extent in every period of human history. However, most historians see the end of the Second World War as a watershed moment.

In 1945, the Western Allies claimed their victory as a victory for freedom. Mass-oriented, collectivist ideologies were declared suspect, not only the defeated Nazi regime but also the new Soviet enemy. The ideology that the United States promoted in opposition to communism (and exported to Europe through the Marshall Plan) was individualism. Personal individualism – the freedom to determine your own destiny – went hand in hand with economic individualism – the freedom to make as much money as you want in order to acquire the lifestyle you want. The pursuit of happiness, asserted in the American Declaration of Independence, seldom came cheap. After digging into reports on prosperity and digesting the relevant graphs and tables, I have reached the conclusion that this economic side of individualism deserves closer scrutiny, as certain economic trends from the second half of the twentieth century have changed not only our view of humanity, but also how we think about fear.

Following a sharp rise in prosperity across most Western European countries in the 1950s, the desire for self-development gained new momentum throughout the 1960s and 1970s. Other lives were within reach: more exciting, more compelling, and free from the interference of narrow-minded paternalism. Suddenly these options became financially available to large numbers of people. Capitalism served this desire, but was also its executor and primary beneficiary. We purchased scooters, cars and plane tickets and travelled the world, everyone an explorer. We were enthralled by the dream of individual fulfilment for all: a new level playing field on which everyone could turn their life around if they so chose. In footballing terms, the West abandoned the lumpy sod of the local common and embraced Astroturf laid out with painstaking precision. In many a European country in the 1990s, this shift became literal as well as metaphorical. At my old club, too, most of the pitches are artificial turf. On hot days, the smell of scorched rubber hangs in the air.

Several philosophers in the 1950s and 1960s warned of the potentially harmful effects of this commodification of happiness. Herbert Marcuse foresaw a world obsessed by money and consumer goods, with a population kept rich, ignorant and antisocial by advertising and relentless technological innovation; a population that would eventually lose the capacity for critical thought. Theodor Adorno believed that the one-dimensionality imposed by capitalism would lead to far-reaching alienation at all levels of society. Sociologist Émile Durkheim referred to this state of increasing disorientation as "anomie". I see alienation, anomie and anxiety as characterisations of the same lonely, disconnected state of being.

Meanwhile, our young footballer in his pink boots sweeps past his first opponent – a quick dummy is enough to leave him standing. Another midfielder slides in with a tackle but misses the mark, thigh scraping across the artificial turf. I wince, remembering the dozens of burning abrasions I suffered as a player: grains of rubber lodged in grazed skin; gritting my teeth as I lowered myself into a hot bath after the game.

We did not become truly anxious until the 1980s, when capitalism shifted gear and took on a new form we now refer to as neo-liberalism: an economic movement in which maximum freedom – and with it, maximum responsibility – was placed in the hands of the individual. Paradoxically, this individualisation brought about a collective change in mentality: economics became integral to the socially accepted ideal of how we should live our lives. At the same time, far from everyone was given the opportunity to live up to that ideal, with anxiety-inducing consequences.

Before I elaborate on the relationship between anxiety and neo-liberalism, it is worth introducing three figures who were central to this transition: Ronald Reagan, US President from 1981 to 1989; Margaret Thatcher, UK Prime Minister from 1979 to 1990, and their chief economic advisor, Milton Friedman.

Let's start with Friedman, who was awarded the Nobel Memorial Prize in Economic Sciences in 1976. Essentially, he was what we now call a free-market fundamentalist. In his view, the only social responsibility a company had was to maximise its profits; by successfully pursuing this goal they were creating benefits for the whole of society, a vision that became more widely known as trickle-down economics. His ideas were adopted by Reagan and Thatcher, two world leaders united by the same ideology. They smashed the power of the trade unions and went on to deregulate the banking sector and virtually every other area of business; the number of people who had to earn a living with little or no collective representation or insurance began to rise. Even in a more collectivist society like the Netherlands, there was a concerted effort by government to stimulate competition in business as much as possible, with an increasing focus on supporting the strong rather than protecting the weak. Former head of Shell Gerrit Wagner summed it up neatly when he said, "Don't back the losers, pick the winners."

Throughout the capitalist West, the age of the shareholder was dawning. Large-scale investors bought up companies, which they then hollowed out with a view to maximising profits. Corporate raiders like these were personified by the character Gordon Gekko played by Michael Douglas in Oliver Stone's 1987 film *Wall Street*. In fact, Gekko's legendary "greed is good" mantra is only a faint echo of what Friedman had been saying all along. "Is there some society you know that doesn't run on greed?" Friedman once asked rhetorically. "What is greed? Of course, none of us are greedy. It's only the other fellow who's greedy. The world runs on individuals pursuing their separate interests." Friedman's ideal was an economy formed by free people engaged in unrestricted competition. This was a system that rewarded traits such as ambition, decisiveness and ruthlessness; other human qualities were merely ballast.

So much for the individual. What about society, the community? "Too many people [. . .] are casting their problems on society," Margaret Thatcher famously said. "And, you know, there is no such thing as society. There are individual men and women and there are families. And no governments can do anything except through people, and people must look after themselves first." Ronald Reagan expressed similar sentiments, for example, in his 1981 inaugural address, when he insisted "Government is not the solution to our problem, government is the problem." The idea seemed to be that if everyone thought of themselves, then everyone would be thought of. "Economics is the method," Mrs Thatcher once said. "The object is to change the soul."

Margaret Thatcher got her way. Our soul did indeed change. Ironically, this change affected our collective soul rather than our individual souls. In the absence of competing ideologies or systems, the market economy gradually led to a market society, to borrow a description from Harvard philosopher Michael Sandel. In concrete terms, this meant that the kind of person you had to be to get ahead in the 1980s and 1990s was fundamentally different from the kind of person you had to be to succeed thirty or forty years previously: the aim was to be highly competitive, to focus on success and status, and to win at all costs. In the market society, trust in others and solidarity were seen as things that usually worked to your disadvantage. This also helped erode our trust in institutions. Whereas in 1964 only 29 per cent of American voters believed that the government was "pretty much run by a few big interests looking out for themselves," by 2013 the view that corruption in government was widespread was held by 79 per cent.

It is important to reflect on the deeper meaning of these shifts. Back in the nineteenth century, the political philosopher John Stuart Mill wrote about economic man as a calculating being who, even when adopting a socially desirable attitude, did so primarily on the basis of self-interest. But in the world that Friedman and Thatcher created, he was expected to have Machiavellian traits too: the more competitive and the more focused on short-term gain economic man was, the more successful he would be. And otherwise, yes, he was a "loser".

Back on the pitch, two defenders still stand between our plucky young striker and his winning goal. Parents roar him on from the sidelines. "Go, go, go! You can do it!" There is the odd premature cry of "Shoot!" The boy's focus seems to narrow.

With all its implications, neoliberalism appears to have had a major impact on how anxious we are. Psychologist and researcher Jean Twenge sees a direct correlation between economic conditions in the post-war Western world and our levels of anxiety. In capitalist systems as we know them in the West, economic value or wealth is a key component of our status and self-esteem. When things get tougher economically, people's self-esteem declines and their anxiety increases. Consequently, the economic crisis of the 1980s immediately triggered a rise in case numbers for depression and anxiety-related conditions. The same thing happened after the 2008 financial crisis, and during the 2020–2021 Covid pandemic.

But hang on a minute: on the whole, aren't we Westerners in a good place economically? What do we have to be afraid of when our standard of living has risen consistently over the years? Well, for one thing, the link between economic conditions and anxiety is not that simple, as evidenced by the extensive work of British social epidemiologist Richard Wilkinson. The key concept is not so much wealth as wealth equality: it's not about the money itself, but an underlying sense of fairness. And the tremendous growth in wealth across the Western world since the Second World War has been distributed anything but evenly.

Take the United States, for example: Will Davies, an economist and sociologist at Goldsmiths College, recently examined developments in the income of US citizens between 1978 and 2015. On average, their income increased by 58 per cent. Good news, you might think. But in real terms, the income of the poorer half of the population had in fact fallen by 1 per cent, while income at the very top – among the richest 0.001 – had risen by 685 per cent. In other words, the 58 per cent average increase in income was severely skewed in ways that only exacerbated the inequality between groups. This is emblematic of a wider picture that holds true for all neoliberal-led countries: a general increase in prosperity is accompanied by a dramatic rise in income inequality.

Since 1990, roughly speaking, the inequality of capital has grown at a remarkable speed, even in more traditionally egalitarian countries such as the Netherlands. This fits seamlessly with French economist Thomas Piketty's assertion that the economic return on wealth is higher and more durable than the return on labour, thereby creating a vicious circle: large disparities in income and wealth lead to greater inequality of opportunity, which in turn results in larger disparities in income and wealth. While Western economies were once sustained by a proletariat, Italian philosopher Paolo Virno argues that today's Western economies are sustained by a growing precariat: a reservoir of working people without financial security, who cannot obtain a mortgage and who, in many cases, do not even know where next month's rent is coming from; people with an exceptionally low "sense of control", who regularly and justifiably fear for their future. We all know someone who belongs to this category: friends and acquaintances who struggle to make ends meet on a monthly basis, sole traders with no collective buffer to fall back on and who feel the immediate impact of every rise in rent.

Richard Wilkinson has shown that countries with large income disparities not only have considerably higher rates of violent crime, drug use and teenage pregnancy than countries with small income disparities but also have a far higher incidence of people with mental health problems. Economics was far from my mind when I set off on this journey, but I have increasingly come to appreciate its relevance to anxiety, thanks to the links Wilkinson demonstrates. It makes sense to me: the more social inequality there is, the more you have to gain or lose, the more important it becomes to beat the competition and the scarier it is when this turns out not to be so easy to achieve. The more you operate on the assumption of equal opportunities or progress, the more devastating it is to see others forging ahead when you are left trailing in their wake. For all its implicit promises and ideals, the modern neoliberal system breeds frustration and fear.

No wonder then, that anxiety disorder should be the most common psychiatric diagnosis in the United States, the ultimate paradise – or hell – of modern capitalism. As already mentioned, official figures for 2017 put the number of adults in the US with an anxiety disorder at approximately 40 million, about 18 per cent of the population. The prevalence is so high that some commentators joke that the country actually has fifty-one states, including the state of anxiety. But in Western European democracies too, the distribution of economic prosperity in recent decades has been far from even, leaving a large group of people feeling marginalised, abandoned, anxious or all of the above. Looking at the specifics: if you are unemployed, you are more than two and a half times more likely to have an anxiety disorder than someone in a paid job. If your income is low, you are almost twice as likely to have an anxiety disorder than someone with an average income. Stress and shame at the prospect of problematic debt lead to fears which may be diagnosed as part of an anxiety disorder. It is worth giving another perspective here too: these are complex statistics, some of which can be turned on their head. Unemployment can lead to anxiety but there are also significant numbers of people who struggle to hold down a steady job because of their battles with anxiety.

Individualism has brought us significant benefits. By giving us more opportunities to develop our talents to the full, it has led to greater personal fulfilment and scientific and technological breakthroughs. The idea that every individual has a right to self-determination and autonomy was also crucial in the rise of civil rights movements and feminist initiatives from the 1960s through the 1980s. But the hyperindividualism that has gone hand in hand with neoliberalism has made us far more psychologically vulnerable than we could ever have imagined.

Our young footballer battles on. One last defender between him and success. His bid for glory revives dim memories of my own hard-fought victories and inglorious defeats, the ferrous smell of grazed skin and the cold slap of a ball heavy with rain. As he charges for goal, I realise that a key piece of the anxiety puzzle is still missing: the reason why the boy in the pink football boots has risen to this challenge. Here, we enter the realm of education and upbringing, more especially the self-esteem movement that emerged in the United States in the mid-1980s and would go on to conquer the entire Western world. This brings us to a Californian politician from the 1980s, as eccentric as he was shady. A Democrat by the name of John 'Vasco' Vasconcellos.

# The Unbearable Legacy of Narcissus

*(Second lesson from the football pitch)*

In his younger years, John Vasconcellos was an altar boy and always on his best behaviour. After serving in the armed forces, he evolved into a politician one reporter described as looking like "a cross between a rock star and a drug smuggler". Vasconcellos was smitten by the work of Carl Rogers, a psychologist who put a quasi-scientific spin on ideas drawn from the immensely popular nineteenth-century New Thought movement and its central concept of positive thinking. Rogers' favourite metaphor was the flower: it needs the right conditions to grow, and starved of nutrition and sunlight, it shrivels and dies. The same is true for us humans, he argued. A person needs a positive environment in which to grow, one that is rooted in openness, empathy, acceptance and even "unconditional positive regard". It's worth letting those words sink in: unconditional positive regard. They signify complete support and acceptance, no matter what choices you make, no matter who you want to become. For years, Rogers' ideas remained confined to academic circles, except for a handful of hippy acolytes in California. It was Vasco the flamboyant politician who freed Rogers from hippiedom and the halls of academe, and unleashed him on the rest of the world.

This occurred in 1986, when Vasco managed to wangle state funding for a three-year task force to assess the value of self-esteem. Vasco's sales pitch was that low self-esteem was the likely cause of countless social problems, from unemployment and substandard education to child abuse and domestic violence. Self-esteem, he argued, was a kind of social panacea. Through a confluence of historical circumstances, the notions of "personal growth" and "finding yourself" were a seamless fit for the times. Self-esteem provided the perfect bridge between the free-thinking ideals of the hippiefied 1960s and 1970s and the prevailing political-economic morale of the 1980s and 1990s, the era of Reagan, Thatcher and their ilk. This bridge offered such a natural way forward that we barely noticed when we had crossed it and reached the other side.

But in September 1988 – by this time Vasco's self-esteem task force was up and running – an academic review of research into self-esteem threatened to burst his bubble. The review's findings painted a contradictory picture: "very positive and compelling" results in some cases, inconclusive or even negative results in others. Having already staked his political reputation on the self-esteem theory, Vasco decided to put the data to creative use. Take, for example, the correlation between higher self-esteem and children who achieved good grades at school. Vasco reversed the law of cause and effect to argue that strong self-esteem was not the result of good grades, as the study had argued, but the cause. Any contradictory or negative results were swept resolutely under the carpet. "I found this was a quasi-religious movement," one academic recalled years later in an interview with journalist Will Storr. A member of Vasco's self-esteem task force put it more bluntly: "It was all a fucking lie."

Task force chairman Andrew Mecca, a confidant of Vasco's, who died in 2014, was soberingly honest when asked about his take on the results. "I didn't care . . . I thought it was beyond science." Vasco and Mecca spent tens of thousands of dollars on a clever PR campaign that enabled them to set and control the narrative.

Mecca was dismissive of those who voiced concerns that data was being distorted. "Who remembers [them]? Nobody! They were tiny ripples in a big tsunami of positive change." But the positivity of that change is open to question. Plenty of scientific research conducted since has shown the link between low self-esteem and poor school performance to be virtually non-existent. In fact, high self-esteem is often an obstacle in dealing with others, associated with a lack of empathy and a notorious inability to realistically assess your own abilities.

Nonetheless, in the newsletter that Vasco and his cohorts drew up a few months later, the "very positive and compelling" side of the story was writ large. This really got the ball rolling. The governor of Arkansas and future US president Bill Clinton got behind the report, as did political heavyweights such as Barbara Bush and Colin Powell. Vasco appeared on talk shows in the US, the UK and Australia. Oprah Winfrey picked up on the movement, stating that self-esteem would become one of the "catch-all phrases for the 1990s". And by saying this on a prime-time television special, she helped make it happen.

The self-esteem movement did indeed bring about a tsunami. Its shock waves fundamentally changed how children in the West were raised. Its ideas found their way into the classroom. In the Netherlands, clinical psychologist Jan Derksen researched this development extensively and in 2009 published a book on what he called "the narcissistic ideal". In the 1980s and 1990s, the children of Western democracies were told that, above all, they should stay true to themselves and love themselves, that they were perfect just as they were and that they could achieve anything they wanted. Advertising slogans made life seem even sweeter. *Impossible is nothing. Because you're worth it. Just do it.* As a result, children were primed to expect more success than their parents had ever known: better jobs, greater recognition, yet more freedom, a life of greater well-being. Yet this culture took root at a time when, in concrete terms, millennials were in considerably worse shape than baby boomers and members of Gen X had been at the same age in terms of pensions, student debt and prospects on the housing market. From the 1980s onwards, the self-determination people had fought for back in the 1960s and 1970s had solidified into a basic attitude, perhaps even a fundamental right. Google tells us that the number of books containing the phrase "you can be anything" increased twelvefold between 1970 and 2008. In 2008, readers were seventeen times more likely to encounter the phrase "follow your dreams" in a book than they had been in 1990, the start of the decade when reality TV took off and fame was dangled within the reach of people being their semi-scripted selves in front of the camera. The phrase "want to be famous" was six times more common in books in 2008 compared to 1960.

I edge closer to the action, toeing the sideline. As the boy in the pink boots closes in on goal, the spectating parents let rip. "Go on! Shoot!" His pace slows. Perhaps, for the first time since launching his one-man offensive, a new thought has flashed through his mind: what if I don't make it?

Virtually all studies looking at the attitudes of today's forty-, thirty- and twenty-somethings reveal them to be significantly more narcissistic than their parents and grandparents were. Narcissism – a term taken from Narcissus, the figure from Greek mythology who fell in love with his reflection – is a trait we all possess to some degree: a mixture of self-esteem and self-confidence, a certain love of self that exists independently of accomplishments or experiences.

Almost all relevant measurements, surveys and reports point to an estimated 30 per cent rise in narcissism in Western societies between 1979 and 2006. We have become more confident in ourselves and less confident in others. Increasingly, we have come to think of ourselves as special or unique. Psychologists and sociologists refer to this increase as the "narcissism epidemic". Narcissism usually comes with an, often unconscious, claim to special treatment and generous helpings of affirmation. This sense of psychological entitlement forms a crucial part of narcissistic personality disorder, a mental health condition catalogued in DSM V, but is also a feature of many of the condescending stereotypes showered on millennials: generation snowflake, spoiled brats, prima donnas, princes and princesses.

From a personal perspective, I recognise these tendencies in myself and my contemporaries, especially when the going gets tough. Not that anyone explicitly insists on their right to be treated a certain way. Entitlement is less about bold statements and more about the questions that surface in response to setbacks and defeats when things refuse to go our way. *What have I done to deserve this? Is this all I have to show for my efforts? How could this happen to someone like me?* Narcissism and entitlement undermine our ability to cope with adversity because they cloud our view of what's really going on. This lack of clear understanding can lead to several kinds of anxiety: panic at feeling overwhelmed, an uneasy sense of failing to grasp how the world works, fear of falling by the wayside. And, underlying it all, that sinking feeling that you're just not good enough.

The narcissistic epidemic has been bad news for society's art of association and the shared norms and values on which it relies. The more members of a group share the dominant norms and values, the stronger their ethical consensus and the stronger the art of association within that group becomes. But thanks to the unstoppable force of individualisation, our notions of morality have become detached from what were once their collective sources: religious texts, shared beliefs and the moral benchmark of the Second World War, fast receding in the rear-view mirror. Cut off from these sources, our moral beliefs, our norms and values, soon proved to be relative and vulnerable. We became moral castaways: still prepared to help the needy, but only once we have found ourselves a serviceable piece of driftwood to cling to. Because we deserve one.

A 2011 study by sociologist Christian Smith, as reported in _The New York Times_ by journalist David Brooks, revealed considerable confusion among young Americans when it comes to moral dilemmas. "When asked to describe a moral dilemma they had faced, two-thirds of the young people either couldn't answer the question or described problems that are not moral at all, like whether they could afford to rent a certain apartment or whether they had enough quarters to feed the meter at a parking spot." So was there no moral basis at all for their actions? "The default position, which most of them came back to again and again, is that moral choices are just a matter of individual taste." As one interviewee said "It's personal. It's up to the individual. Who am I to say?" Another responded "I would do what I thought made me happy . . . I have no other way of knowing what to do but how I internally feel."

Smith's findings about collective moral disorientation also hold true in Europe. According to figures published by the Institute for Social Research in the Netherlands, the percentage of Dutch people who thought norms and values had deteriorated rose from forty to sixty per cent between 1968 and 2006, peaking in 1998, when seventy per cent believed there had been a moral decline. The respondents also expressed growing doubts about their own moral judgement. In 2008, forty per cent of Dutch people between the ages of 21 and 64 agreed with the statement: "Everything changes so quickly these days, it's often hard to tell right from wrong." This was the highest percentage in almost 30 years.

Back on the pitch, the last defender makes his move. Our striker checks, stumbles, but keeps possession and is back on his way. Shaking off all hesitation, he pours everything he has into one final burst of speed. Now it's just him and the keeper. His dream of scoring that winning goal is in sight. Just do it.

*

The myth of Narcissus has always intrigued me. Not because he fell in love with his own reflection, but because he kept on looking until he died. To me, there is a cruel wisdom in that fate. Just as Narcissus succumbed to the unbridgeable gap between reflection and reality, many young people in the 1980s and 1990s foundered in the face of an unbridgeable gap between expectation and reality. Attempts have been made to adjust reality to fit expectations, as evidenced by the tendency towards grade inflation at schools and colleges. In the United States, the percentage of students who achieved an A average in high school rose from 18 to 48 per cent between the 1960s and 2004, while the results of SATs (standardised university admissions tests) suggested that standards had in fact declined. Teachers at one British school began marking homework in mauve instead of red ink so as not to upset their pupils. At some US schools, kids were given a trophy simply for turning up for sports day.

If adjustment fails to ease the pain, there is always evasion. An interesting psychological escape for today's narcissistically inclined human is gaming, a culture and an industry that gathered steam from around 1990. Where people used to play games together, with cards, dice or pieces on a board, we can now sit alone on the couch and dive into all manner of digital fantasy worlds. This change in how we play is partly driven by technological advances, of course, but it also stems from a desire deep within us. It is now possible to dispense with other players in the real world and inhabit the role of the one true hero in a fantasy world with the power to alter the course of events: a narcissistic fantasy, a sense of ultimate control. It is no accident that a growing number of films and TV shows focus on the theme of choosing imaginary worlds over the physical world we inhabit: *The Matrix* (1999), *Avatar* (2009), *Ready Player One* (2018), *Black Mirror* (2011–present) and *Maniac* (2018).

But evasions and stopgaps designed to cushion the comedown from the heady brew on which we were raised (capitalism as ideology + social engineering as the dream + self-fulfilment as the ideal + high self-esteem as a basic belief) cannot shield us from life's fundamental lesson for ever: that the playing field is anything but level. Setbacks and opposition are built into the game. Skin colour, background, age, gender, class, the degree of talent and discipline you possess, not to mention blind luck, all have their effect on your career and the course of your life. We have struggled and failed to reconcile this practical wisdom, an insight taken for granted for centuries, with the individualistic illusions that informed our upbringing.

"We live in a culture of success," psychiatrist Jan Swinkels explains. "People aren't given the time to mature or to learn anymore. You only learn by making mistakes, but make one mistake and you can be out on your ear. There are only a few people who truly succeed, while the rest of us are made to feel like losers. Our fixation on success and our compulsion to classify every problem as a mental health problem leave many people feeling unsafe, unprotected, unhealthy." Swinkels argues that, as human beings, we work towards two interrelated goals. "The first is autonomy: being able to make your own decisions about your life. The second is contact with others and being treated humanely in that context. And when those needs are frustrated, we become angry or anxious."

Young people in the 1980s, 1990s and beyond discovered that what they had learned about life was completely out of sync with the world around them. This inevitably led to inner conflict. To quote one anxiety-fuelled text message I recently received – the time stamp of four in the morning suggested a difficult night – *They always say that every individual is responsible for their own life. But what do you do when it's not the life you want?* When human wisdom reached a point where the primal forces of chance, chaos or divine retribution no longer counted as an acceptable explanation, the blame for every setback came to lie with us. And in this binary success-or-failure mindset where shades of grey reek of failure, the chance of seeing yourself as a loser is many times higher than the chance of being content with what you have.

The short circuit created by this colossal mismatch between expectation and reality has led to a dramatic increase in helplessness, anxiety and frustration, which in turn has prompted an unprecedented rise in psychiatric disorders throughout the Western world. The trade in labels and drugs, which fits the economic and individualistic zeitgeist like a glove, has grown accordingly. But this system also met a major psychological need of the time: the conferral of a psychiatric label relieved us of our sense of responsibility, at least for a while. It wasn't our fault that we couldn't keep up with the pace of modern-day existence, it was because of our illness. And all the while our fear and anger were growing.

"Never have we been so free. Never have we felt so powerless." A neater summary of our predicament than the one provided by Polish-British sociologist Zygmunt Bauman is hard to come by. Especially when you consider that powerlessness and anxiety are closely linked. In the end, many fears come down to an inability to cope with anxiety. Agoraphobia, for instance, can be seen as the fear of being overwhelmed by fear in public, and panic as the fear of being overwhelmed by a feeling (in most cases anxiety). Generalised anxiety, meanwhile, can be put down to an ever-present doubt about being able to withstand the challenges life throws at us.

One way of obtaining an accurate picture of our struggles is by looking at the slogans attached to the health hypes that come our way. The emphasis that yoga and mindfulness place on learning to let go shows us how much importance we attach to control. "Anxiety is essentially feeling a lack of control," psychiatrist Damiaan Denys tells me. "Control over the outside world, your inner world, your thoughts and your loved ones. We seek to compensate by working frantically to gain control of ourselves and the outside world. But to genuinely counteract our fears, we need to relinquish our need for control and accept that things don't always go the way we want them to, that we cannot control everything. This mental shift has become very hard for us to achieve, enabling fear to spiral from an individual emotion into a social phenomenon."

The pieces of the puzzle are falling into place. Almost enough to provide a tentative answer to the seemingly simple question of why we have become more afraid. One more piece to go.

Tantalisingly close. Exactly what our pink-booted footballer must be thinking. With only a few more yards to go, he is poised to strike, to seize his moment. Then, out of nowhere, one final challenge. A midfielder has charged back and lunges at the ball with a well-timed tackle. The striker is thrown off balance, loses his footing, falls. No whistle from the referee. Desperate, silent seconds follow. Our would-be hero looks around, dazed and shattered. What now?

# 12

# Crossed Lines

*(Third lesson from the football pitch)*

Incandescent with rage, the parents of the felled striker turn on the referee: the parents of a ten-year-old boy spit venom at a middle-aged man in an oversized windbreaker who, in exchange for a toasted sandwich and a mug of tea, has sacrificed a chunk of his Saturday to officiate at a kids' football match. This riles the parents of the tackler, who start mouthing off at the striker's parents. Everyone on and around the field seems to erupt with pent-up frustration. Pandemonium ensues. The referee calls it a day, blows an impromptu final whistle and high-tails it off the pitch. Is it a draw or has the match been forfeited? No-one knows.

As my thoughts drift from education to philosophy, it occurs to me that this is not an isolated case. All over the world, supposedly impartial bodies, those who set the boundaries of the permissible, from art experts to broadcasters and from judges to referees, are coming under intense pressure. Players and parents alike bicker about the referee and his supposed lack of judgement, about which team was robbed. But where does the truth lie? Who has the answer?

My gaze swings skywards to the birds circling high above the Astroturf. Disheartened by the chaotic end to the match, and bewildered as to how a simple tackle could unleash such pandemonium, I take a deep breath and close my eyes. I try to picture that most enviable of vantage points, a bird's eye view. My fingers reach instinctively for something to hold on to and grasp the phone in my pocket. (Batman has replaced D. as my screensaver.) I open my eyes.

In addition to our lost art of association, another recent development has undermined our grip on reality. Western societies are dealing with what French philosopher François Ewald has described as a crisis of causality: we are no longer able to see the causal relationship between actions and consequences. This relatively new phenomenon cannot be separated from the unprecedented increase in information available to one and all thanks to the internet. In the seventeenth century, the age in which our modern belief in reason and objective knowledge took shape, Thomas Hobbes – no stranger to anxiety himself   concluded his political-philosophical masterpiece *Leviathan* (1651) with the immortal lines: "For such Truth, as opposeth no man's profit, nor pleasure, is to all men welcome." Universal Truth as a universal antidote.

What was the nature of this truth to which Hobbes laid claim in his great work? It was a construct of arguments, logic and irrefutable conclusions. Almost a century later, philosopher Denis Diderot completed the Herculean task of producing his *Encyclopédie* (1751–1772), a vastly ambitious tome in which he provided explanations for every worldly phenomenon, in the hope that greater knowledge would lead to greater happiness. His assumption: if we all had access to the same facts, we would have no choice but to agree and happiness would surely be within reach.

Such thinking was revolutionary at the time. Today, it strikes us as naive. We know all too well that information is distinct from knowledge, and no-one would be so presumptuous as to capitalise the word truth, never mind stick the word universal in front of it. The idea that one truth fits all has felt hopelessly outdated since the advent of postmodernism. For every conceivable proposition, every conceivable "truth", a reservoir of supporting "evidence" can be found online. The same applies to each opposing position. We live in an impenetrable and complex world, without much in the way of factual guidance. For anxiety, there is no better breeding ground imaginable.

This chaotic lack of clarity also partly explains the gulf that exists in the Western world between safety as it is measured and as it is perceived. Although official figures tell us that our lives are becoming ever safer, we feel increasingly unsafe. For over seventy years we have not experienced a major conflict in Western Europe, but we do not feel at peace. Crime rates in the US and the UK have been falling for years, yet there is a widespread perception that crime is on the rise. Even in the Netherlands, where the gap between safety and perceived safety is traditionally small, 54 per cent of the population believe crime is increasing, though this is by no means the case. This is sometimes referred to as the fear paradox: in a world that is safer than ever, we are more fearful than ever. That has always struck me as a simplistic view. As we have already seen, there are many areas in which the world has actually become much more unsafe within a relatively short time span – economically, ecologically, geopolitically and therefore psychologically. Physical safety is only a very small part of what allows someone to feel safe. In the absence of physical threats such as war and hunger, fears and frustrations still have the power to work their way under our skin and infiltrate our inner world.

The media reinforce these tendencies. Reports on crime and disasters beyond our control are much more frequent than they used to be, collectively saddling us with feelings of helplessness or even despair. There is a strong correlation between media consumption and feeling unsafe: the more news you watch and read, the more unsafe you tend to feel. "There are fewer terrorist attacks in Europe today than there were in the 1970s and 1980s, yet you read and hear far more about terrorism than you did then," Damiaan Denys observes. "Newspapers want to sell copies, TV shows crave ratings, and negative news has more pulling power than positive news. But it's not just the media that play on our fears; businesses do it too. Commercials used to be about whisky and cigarettes. About a more sophisticated, more luxurious lifestyle. Later the message became: you can be anything you want to be. But increasingly, the message is changing to: you have no idea how much danger you are in. Ads for toiletries to combat body odour you can't smell yourself. For cleaning products that battle invisible germs. For cars that brake automatically, in case you've overlooked something or someone. Growing up in this kind of media environment, you incorporate anxiety into your outlook."

We can now conclude that Hobbes and Diderot were wrong in this respect: truth and knowledge have not made us happy; nor have they cured us or liberated us from uncertainty and fear. In fact, leading sociologists such as Ulrich Beck and Anthony Giddens have argued convincingly that the global increase in knowledge resulting from the scientific revolution and the subsequent digital revolution have led to a collective sense of insecurity. Beck even goes one step further, arguing that the primary source of danger is no longer ignorance, as we have assumed for centuries, but knowledge. Who is right? Everyone. No-one.

In this context, it is also worth talking about the thing I instinctively reached for as all hell broke loose around me – my phone. The smartphone only entered our lives in 2007, but it has significantly ramped up the wider developments outlined in this chapter, amplifying narcissism and diluting connectedness. Yet in the early days of online communication, the possibilities offered by a telephone with easy internet access were warmly welcomed. Digital utopians predicted that this new technology would expand and enrich our social contacts, bringing people together across vast distances, day or night. Distinctions based on gender, ethnicity, disability or socioeconomic background would become less of an issue.

Years later, the scientific consensus is considerably more grim:

online communication appears to create an accumulation of advantages rather than a fairer distribution. In other words, it enhances social contact for those who already have rich social lives. While there are examples of socially anxious and lonely young people who dare to engage more with others in the digital world than they do in the physical world, all too often their online contact echoes their negative experiences in real life. Scientists speak of the Matthew effect: the haves flourish on the basis of their existing advantages, while those who have less fall further behind. Technologically speaking, there has never been a time in human history when it has been as easy to connect with others as it is today. Yet that digital contact is often accompanied by physical loneliness. And while the likes of Facebook, Twitter and Instagram have become part of our modern lives and do generate moments of happiness and connection, studies show that they often bring frustration, anxiety and feelings of inadequacy or even failure.

There are several reasons for this. One is that they have made popularity measurable: everyone can see how many people like you. The more people like you, the more likes you get, and the more friends or followers you attract. The more followers you have, the easier it is to gain new followers, thanks to the nature of the underlying algorithms developed by the billion-dollar companies behind these platforms. Popularity breeds popularity. Implicitly, the opposite also applies: unpopularity increases the likelihood of remaining unpopular.

Then there is the neurochemical component of our attachment to this technology: each like triggers the release of hormones that boost our alertness, such as adrenaline and dopamine. Dopamine in particular is a pleasurable and addictive hormone, one which – contrary to popular belief – relates primarily to the expectation of reward rather than to pleasure itself. Our phones bring that expectation into sharp relief, tapping into our deep-seated need to be seen and feel appreciated. "Every like is a moment of self-affirmation," as internet pioneer Marleen Stikker puts it. But perhaps the description provided by my fellow fearty P. makes the point even better: "When I get a like, it means someone somewhere in the world is thinking of me at that very moment." The line between virtual applause and existential affirmation is extremely thin. Which explains the humiliation we feel when we share something important to us and receive only a handful of likes in response. And why cyberbullying often has such a devastating impact.

Another aspect is the rose-tinted effect that kicks in when we look around online and see enhanced versions of other people's lives, in stark contrast to our own. The photos people post invite us to focus on their success and happiness, while a flattering shot of yourself comes with a backstory: yesterday, it was all I could do to drag myself out of bed. Other people's happiness often appears so much more convincing or self-evident than our own, perhaps because a throwaway moment of romantic bliss from another life looks like a single frame from an endless stream of equally blissful moments, while our own happy snaps remind us how awkward we felt posing for them. The online image of others, often so naturally appealing, sets a standard that our own messy lives can only fail to live up to. Without realising it, we subject ourselves to dozens of hopeless comparison contests on a daily basis, in which the worst version of ourselves does battle with the best version of other people, contests with plenty of losers and no real winner. Social media can breed envy and plant seeds of inferiority, seeds that may or may not grow into anxiety or depression.

The extent of our smartphone addiction is especially apparent among young people. In 2015, over 70 per cent of Western teens had access to a smartphone, an estimate that has surely gone up since. The number of American high school students aged fourteen to sixteen who struggle with loneliness increased by 31 per cent between 2012 and 2015. And in 2015, 56 per cent more teens experienced depression than in 2010. Young people who have grown up with smartphones have relatively little social contact: they go to fewer parties and see their friends less regularly than young people from earlier generations. Virtually every study on the effects of social media concludes that there is a direct link between screen time and feeling anxious or depressed.

Our would-be football hero has dusted himself down and wanders off the pitch to ask his dad if they can go home now. On closer inspection, his pink boots bear Cristiano Ronaldo's CR7 logo. When he reaches the threshold age of 13, he will doubtless join the ranks of Ronaldo's 150 million Instagram followers. Unconsciously, I, the boy, all of us see the image celebrities project on Instagram as evidence of their fame or happiness. If we succeed in recreating the elements of that image – the exclusive locations, the designer shades, the sleek yacht in the background – doesn't that make us successful? "We know what we are, but know not what we may be," Ophelia says in *Hamlet*. Our online fixations turn this on its head: we know exactly what we may be, yet struggle to see what we actually are.

Of course, there is no point in overlooking the enjoyment, entertainment and connection that social media bring most of us on a daily basis. But as the months and the years add up, the balance tips in an unfortunate direction, reinforcing and aggravating our narcissistic tendencies, with all the pitfalls and drawbacks that entails.

A dull thud and a piercing wail snap me back to full alertness. A ball lobbed over the fence by a player on pitch No. 3 has bounced off a parked car. The sound of the alarm echoes around the surrounding buildings. Sobered by the game and perhaps a little misty-eyed from my own vague memories of Saturday afternoons spent running around here as a kid, I leave the pitch as the stragglers head for the changing rooms. Two new teams are already itching to take their place, the Astroturf beckons. The parents head up to the cafeteria for a plate of meatballs or a cheese roll. I trudge along behind them as the clouds close in. There's rain on the way.

What can I take away from this visit to my old club? What has it told me about the observation that people in the West have grown more fearful since the 1980s? I saw a young boy detach himself from the team, expectantly chasing his moment to shine. I looked on as his charge for glory hit the outstretched leg of an opponent, a tackle that sparked a furious, chaotic response. Watching, I pondered weighty words and complex theories, dropped a few resounding names: disorienting, perhaps, to wend our way through so many different fields of study that are usually viewed in isolation. But as I see it, they all feed into the bigger picture. How can we get to grips with the world if we are blinded by borders?

The birth – or rather, the creation – of our modern-day *homo anxiosus* is not the product of a masterplan or a revolution. Instead, he has emerged from a succession of wider processes, seemingly unrelated events and developments that have become linked in a unique chain of action and reaction. Compare it to the Earth's surface, formed by the slow shifting of tectonic plates, gigantic suboceanic and subterranean plateaus that happened to collide, resulting in the mountains and valleys we take for granted today.

What tectonic movements have resulted in *homo anxiosus* and his entry into the regime of the DSM? Our insatiable desire for greater individual freedom has robbed us of the ability to cope with our fears collectively, in communities or associations, with or without a belief in God. From a position of solidarity, we have gravitated towards a more solitary existence. At the same time, a process of erosion took place and our traditional ways of dealing with our fears lost their power. Our surrender to capitalism not only led to the propagation of the American dream of freedom, it also created huge disparities between rich and poor, which in turn have impacted on our fears. Either consciously or unconsciously, figures like Margaret Thatcher, Ronald Reagan and even a curious second-rate politician like John Vasconcellos helped to fuse economics with identity. The insidious influence of the self-esteem movement has left us feeling lonelier and more narcissistic. The advent of the internet brought us plenty of positives, but has also gone on to further erode the concept of truth. And then there has been the rise of psychopharmaceuticals, providing an escape for many when the feelings of inadequacy became too intense to bear. (This summary is not to rule out the possibility that other developments have also played their part, albeit less markedly.)

I am not out to label one historical development good and another bad. They are simply developments with consequences – both direct and indirect – which can sometimes take decades to digest. Identifying these consequences does not represent a veiled plea for conservatism or a nostalgic longing for the way things were. On the whole, you can say that something is lost and something gained in every era, and there is often a direct relationship between the two. What have we won in the last fifty years? Individual freedom and greater equality. What have we lost? A sense of belonging. Something to hold on to. What has enriched us? New ways of communicating with others. What has slipped away? Our ability to connect. What have we cultivated? Self-esteem. What have we overlooked? Humility. What have we gained in abundance? Information. What have we lost? A sense of perspective.

All these processes have created a world in which human anxiety could flourish. Never before have so many people been so scared. Growing up in this day and age has had an undeniably powerful influence on our anxiety. The time in which you grow up accounts for an estimated twenty per cent of the difference in anxiety levels across generations. In practical terms, you can grow up in a stable, loving family and nevertheless experience heightened anxiety simply because you are living here and now.

The time has come to leave behind the overarching story of fear and its causes and effects for a while and return to the one story only I can tell: my own. Heading for the green gate, I pass the dead zone where I once heard Japie's mocking voice: "Ha! Lard Arse!" The rack is a jumble of bikes, not so much parked as thrown together.

Dented cans of energy drink litter the pavement and black specks of Astroturf rubber clog the grooves between the slabs. As a young boy, crushed by Japie's putdown, I tried to write him a letter. There were two versions. The first was pure rage, in the second I tried to understand him. I wrote them knowing they would never leave the confines of my diary. They went unsent, but I kept on writing. Because there was something more important than being heard.

# Intermezzo

## *O Fear, I Know Thee*

For days after my visit to the football club, having laid out the puzzle of *homo anxiosus*, I have to make a conscious effort to shake off the spectre of Japie. His slick, black hair, his freckled cheeks, his mocking smirk. My childhood diaries are untraceable; I have to make do with memories, which haunt me like they used to. A wide-eyed little boy stares at me from the mirror, puzzled by the lines around his eyes. When I confided in D. about the child I once was, she fantasised about travelling back in time to ruffle my hair and ask me out on a future date; a prospect to cling to when times got rough.

As I rattle around the apartment, reflections and memories take over. Of the parties we threw here. How we sized up our outfits beforehand, chuckling at each other's fashion risks ("Tiger print? Who are you going as – J.Lo?") How we celebrated her graduation, the publication of my latest book. We moved in together in 2017, uncharted territory for both of us. Fuelled by ham sandwiches fresh from the baker's on what was now our street, we whitewashed walls and sawed planks into shelves. Shoulder to shoulder, we restructured our love lives until all the one-night stands, doe-eyed infatuations and fledgling relationships had become a prelude to the story we were shaping together, sometimes with weighty words but mostly with simple deeds. Popping down to the baker's on a Saturday and ordering for each other. Becoming regulars at a local restaurant, where they scrawled our names on the paper tablecloths, with an exclamation mark for good measure.

I wander from room to room, plucking books from the shelves. It's only when I sit down to read that my composure returns. Poetry works well, especially when I feel alienated, clutching at words to describe (or legitimise) my mood.

It doesn't take me long to settle on the Romantics. John Keats' "Ode on Melancholy" (1819) which urges us, above all else, to remain melancholy, to embrace bouts of sadness and fear as they fall "sudden from heaven like a weeping cloud". Clouds are not only dark and terrifying, but also nourishing and vital. William Collins in his "Ode to Fear" (1746) took a similar view, writing "O fear, I know thee by my throbbing heart". Collins thought that fear could be a guide, the same spirit that drove Shakespeare to write his finest work. He ends with the words "And I, O fear, will dwell with thee!" Perhaps, instead of dissecting the damage fear can do and the hold it has over us, it is time to dwell on what it has brought us; the letters written by fear, the ideas it has shaped, and even the works of art it has generated.

I scribble the odd note: jumbled fragments – a bunch of flowers, a kitchen conversation. Scraps and scrawls, practically unreadable, which will one day result in this book's opening chapter. I read on, drifting from cover to cover.

Until I light on a little red book, one I haven't thought about in a long time. *Fears of Your Life* was written by a man called Michael Bernard Loggins. The author information on the back flap is sketchy. But it gives me a place to start. San Francisco.

# 13

# The Curious Case of
# Michael Bernard Loggins

The Golden Gate Bridge, San Francisco. A suitcase heavy with Romantic poetry and scholarly articles. Slotted in among the books, cushioned by a layer of shirts and socks, is a print of Edvard Munch's *Anxiety*, a painting from 1894 and part of the *Frieze of Life* series in which he depicted fear of every kind, not least the anguish of his best-known work *The Scream*. The print is a gift for Michael Bernard Loggins, an African-American outsider artist who in 2004 published a long list of his fears, a work of art in book form. Fear has taken such a toll on Michael's life that his work will probably never reach a wide audience. But it asks fascinating questions about the line between genius and madness. How many fears can you have before they turn against you and your work?

Connecting with Michael proves to be no mean feat. He has no email address of his own. The small publishing house that produced his book *Fears of Your Life* puts me in touch with two go-betweens: the owner of the workshop-cum-art-studio Michael visits from time to time, and his health advisor. They know where Michael lives, but warn me that my chances of finding him there are slim. Instead, they recommend hanging out in a little park that he frequents. I spend days bench-sitting, all to no avail.

The workshop owner reckons it would be a good idea to buy a few more gifts to add to my print and tells me that Michael is into vinyl: old 45s in particular. I browse the racks at a bunch of shabby record stores and come away with a cache of vintage tunes. And just when I'm starting to wonder what the hell I think I'm doing, fate intervenes. The health advisor calls with good news of sorts: Michael has had surgery on his foot and is in no shape to roam the city streets. And so on a sun-drenched Californian Friday, I head over to visit him at the assisted living unit he occupies in the heart of what used to be hippy central, where even today hundreds of homeless people in garbage-bag ponchos sing songs about beating the system.

Michael lives in a room about sixteen feet by twenty, much of which is taken up with crates of records and endless piles of clothes. A plastic Christmas tree and a supermarket trolley stuffed with yet more clothes complete the scene. Michael is lying on his bed, one foot bandaged, wearing checked pyjama bottoms and no top. A message for the surgeon is written in black marker on his right shin: *It's this leg!*

The first of my 45s break the ice and he gets me to spin them right away. Aretha Franklin, followed by Howlin' Wolf. As the music plays, Michael passes comment, but it takes me a while to tune in to his voice. He is missing several teeth, smacks his lips when he talks and has a tendency to free associate. His conversation is peppered with words of his own making: these include *blue out* (a milder version of a blackout), *dramaticalisms* (instances of dramatic behaviour), *humanful* (kind, considerate), and my particular favourite *clownsmenship* (the camaraderie between a group of clowns).

During our first encounter, he bombards me with questions. Each one feels like a test. Some even sound like riddles: "How old were you when you were young?" Or "What do you like best: the cash you pay for lemonade or for girl scout cookies?" I rely on wild guesswork but know instantly when I get an answer wrong.

Michael's face never keeps you guessing: when he is happy, he smiles with everything he's got and when he's not, his face creases up in disgust. Words are precious to him. If we don't know what words mean, he explains, how can we ever talk to each other? He is on a constant search for the right shade of meaning, a quest he calls "taming the world". Before I leave, he gets me to help him to the toilet. His hand is limp and clammy. The trust he puts in me is pure and complete, a level of trust that must have caused him all kinds of pain.

Two days later, I'm back with another peace offering: cheese-burgers this time. His mind is clearer today and memories come thick and fast, though they remain jumbled. Michael leaps back and forth through his life story. It begins in 1961, when he was born into a family of nine children in San Francisco. As a new-born, he was consigned to an incubator for a time, and a childhood dogged by thyroid problems left him unable to speak. All he could do was point, howl and cause a ruckus. The family moved from house to house, never putting down roots. His parents called him Michael, he explains, because the name doesn't run in the family – a typical example of Loggins logic. He started to write at the age of three, simply because he couldn't talk. So what did he write about? "Things that happened to me, that I didn't understand. Things that were suddenly gone. Things that hurt." Michael would draw and write at his parents' kitchen table, often for hours on end. "It made me happy, and that really surprised my mother. And I wanted to get better at it. And then I actually got good at it. My thoughts move very quickly when I'm working, they shoot past on every side. When Michael Bernard Loggins writes," he declares, "he's like a real person." I wonder what he means. Did writing about his pain make him feel more human?

Since the days of ancient Greece, artists have been open about their mental instability, often interpreting it as an expression of melancholy, a state of being that has occupied a special place in the world of illness: as a precursor to depression and overwhelming anxiety, but also as a precondition for genius. "Madness, provided it comes as the gift of heaven, is the channel by which we receive the greatest blessings," Socrates is quoted as saying, "[A] nobler thing than sober sense [. . .] madness comes from God, whereas sober sense is merely human." He went on to say that the work of the artist who has not been touched by divine madness, who thinks they can get by on technique alone, will always be eclipsed by the achievements of the inspired madman.

Following this line of reasoning, Aristotle asked in his highly influential work *Problems*, "Why is it that all men who are outstanding in philosophy, poetry or the arts are melancholic?" In his view, the answer was to be found in the unique mixing ratio of black bile to other bodily fluids, or humours as they were known. This balance was a precarious one; if it was upset, the melancholic could be plunged into strange or excessive behaviour. By the end of his book, Aristotle even turns the bold statement above on its head, claiming that all melancholics are exceptional. In doing so, he offers an indirect response to Socrates: divine madness and melancholy are one and the same.

Artists of all countries, eras and disciplines have talked about their inner pain as integral to their work. Beethoven declared melancholy to be his muse and Friedrich Schiller maintained that we are all melancholy. Edgar Allan Poe wrote about falling in love with melancholy, Virginia Woolf saw it as her most powerful inspiration and Van Gogh observed that the more spent and ill he was, the more of an artist he became. Joni Mitchell said depression can be "the sand that makes the pearl", John Cale sang that fear was man's best friend, Edvard Munch called his "fear of life" the rudder of his ship. "My art is grounded in being different from others," he said. "My sufferings are part of myself and my art [. . .] I want to keep those sufferings." The refrain of one of the Dutch writer Joost Zwagerman's poems runs: "Afraid of it all. Always afraid of it all.

T.S. Eliot took a different view of the direct and striking relationship between fear and inspiration. One of the 20th century's seminal poets, Eliot did not see inspiration as a positive force rising from within but as the falling away of limitations. "To me," he wrote, "it seems that at these moments, which are characterised by the sudden lifting of the burden of anxiety and fear which presses upon our daily life so steadily that we are unaware of it, what happens is something *negative*: that is to say, not 'inspiration' as we commonly think of it, but the breaking down of strong habitual barriers."

An impressive roll-call of names that mean little or nothing to Michael.

That evening, in my hotel room, I dip into the scientific works I have brought with me and am reminded that the madness associated with so many great artists runs far deeper than a melodramatic martyr complex. In 1972, psychologist Colin Martindale published a survey of the lives of twenty-one British and twenty-one French poets of note. He concluded that over 55 per cent of the British and 40 per cent of the French poets had a history of serious mental illness, as evidenced by nervous breakdowns, psychotic episodes, alcoholism, admissions to psychiatric wards and suicide. The corresponding rate in the general population at the time lay between 1 and 2 per cent.

Another interesting study was carried out by psychiatrist Arnold Ludwig, who examined the biographies of artists whose work had been discussed in *The New York Times Book Review* between 1960 and 1990. Ludwig found that artists who fitted this profile were two to three times more likely to experience mental health problems than non-artists. The likelihood of their being involuntarily admitted to psychiatric care was six to seven times higher. But perhaps the most extensive study was conducted by psychiatrist Kay Redfield Jamison. In 1993, Jamison studied all the major British and Irish poets born between 1705 and 1805. She read their work, delved into their medical records, picked her way through their letters and sifted through observations jotted down by their contemporaries. She found that, for these poets, the likelihood of being committed to psychiatric care was twenty times that of the general population. More than half the poets suffered from mood swings, and their risk of manic depression was over thirty times higher than the average. Today, she concluded, most of the Romantic poets of eighteenth-century Britain would probably be in line for psychiatric treatment. Samuel Johnson regularly suffered breakdowns throughout his life; he had tics, obsessions, phobias, and saw himself as a chronic melancholic. The modern diagnosis would probably be depression. Robert Burns was affected by seasonal melancholy he described as "groaning under the miseries of a diseased nervous system". The likely modern diagnosis: bipolar disorder. The same applies to William Wordsworth, Lord Byron, John Keats and Samuel Taylor Coleridge, with his outspoken references to the melancholy and anxiety that tormented him but were also the flames that kept his inner poet alive. "We of the craft are all crazy," Byron concluded. "Some are affected by gaiety, others by melancholy, but all are more or less touched."

Studies of living writers show a similar pattern. Neuroscientist Nancy Andreasen examined participants in the Iowa Writers' Workshop and found that the percentage of writers who met the formal criteria for a mood disorder was nearly three times higher than the average. No matter which study I pick up, the results are more or less the same: statistically speaking, an artistic profession of any kind appears to be fraught with danger, possibly even up there with soldier or snake charmer.

So how does this "madness" transmute into art?

From a neurological perspective, there appear to be two aspects to this connection: one is flexibility and speed of thought, the other is the ability to combine those thoughts. People in a hypomanic state excel in both these areas, my reading reveals. Hypomania is a condition of intense excitement that sometimes precedes mania.

In modern-day parlance it is often referred to as "flow". Enter a flow state and you become mentally detached from what is going on around you, oblivious to time and place. A brain scan would reveal multiple areas of enhanced activity in both hemispheres of the brain. In a flow state, you have a relatively large number of thoughts within a given time and they come at a faster rate, sometimes shooting off in all directions. This is accompanied by a heightened sensitivity, not only to what others experience, but also to what you are feeling and thinking yourself. Functioning at a higher intellectual level, you are quick to hit upon the words, images, ideas and associations you need, free to riff and improvise, and much more besides. This greater freedom enables you to mix, match and combine with effortless assurance. Unfettered by boundaries or categories, liberated from the need to home in on a particular answer or end point, a playful sense of adventure takes you wherever the flow may lead. This relatively chaotic state of mind, which usually lasts a few hours, produces constant collisions and cross-pollinations. Then, as the flow subsides, you gradually come back down to earth, often feeling a little drained. If, instead of ebbing away, the intensity of the flow continues to build, you can be propelled into a state of mania. Or, if delusions arise and order does not reassert itself, the next phase is psychosis.

What about the periods of depression, melancholy and anxiety? What purpose do they serve? They are calmer and generate little in the way of energy. The storm of ideas has abated and such periods can offer a chance to put those ideas into some kind of perspective. Rather than being overconfident, the melancholic, depressed or anxious artist is racked with doubt, afraid of making something bad, afraid of what others might think. Their caution, their fear, keeps them from making mistakes. The melancholic, depressed or anxious artist looks back on life, and in doing so is able to draw on impressions from any number of troubling episodes that would otherwise have been repressed or shoved aside.

Michael, too, is one of the melancholy, though it's not a term he would ever use. He appears to thinks differently from most of us, investing words with new meanings to construct an original and sometimes mysterious vocabulary all of his own. Though it's hard to be sure, his experience of the world appears to differ profoundly from mine. Perhaps a hint of this can be found in how he responds to his memories. The sudden recollection of someone not wanting to sit next to him on the bus can send him into a tailspin, while he rarely gives a thought to far more harrowing events from his teenage years. He lived with his parents until they died a few years ago in quick succession, but their deaths upset him less than a hurtful comment made in 1992 by someone he took to be his friend; it is the way of things for parents to pass on, but that friend had betrayed his trust.

His fears operate in much the same way: Michael's developmental disability leads him to assign them all equal weight. Fear No. 50 in *Fears of Your Life* (fear of being spanked by a schoolteacher who has got your parents' permission to do so) is as crushing as No. 27 (fear of getting left alone) or No. 51 (fear of sexual abuse). No. 53 (fear of bats) hurts just as much as No. 57 (fear of being different). And No. 87 (fear of getting hugged by somebody you don't like) is as hard to brush aside as No. 98 (fear of people who are scared of Michael).

It is the complete absence of hierarchy that makes his list of fears so powerful. Both extraordinary and disarming, it highlights how many perceived dangers surround us on any given day, the arbitrary nature of our distinction between rational and irrational fears, and the fragility of our sense of security. Michael's most pressing fears this week are that the chicken pot pie he has for breakfast will burn away his intestines, and that the television will fall over and kill him with a surge of electricity. Michael Bernard Loggins lives a life without filters.

One major difference between Michael and the artists mentioned earlier in this chapter is his conviction that fear has brought him nothing good. On my second visit, I try to convince him that without his fears he might never have written or drawn anything and that his book of fears would certainly never have existed – fear as a curse and a source of inspiration. Michael just shrugs.

Can he remember a day when he was not afraid?

He shakes his head. And if he wasn't afraid, then he was afraid of being afraid, a sense of foreboding that put him on edge, and left him feeling jittery and insecure.

Where does he feel this fear?

He clasps his belly. "In Michael Bernard Loggins's gut."

What is fear to him?

"Fear is like a car coming straight at you and you can't stop it, and you can't step aside either, and you're probably wearing the wrong kind of shoes, and so you fall. You're always falling."

Why did he decide to write down all his fears?

"To understand what they mean. What fear can do to you. You got to understand fear and learn from it. Otherwise you hurt people. There's no other way. You can try to hide fear, like a dog hides a bone. But then someone else finds the bone, and he'll beat you with it."

At the end of our third meeting – a triple whammy of 45s, cheeseburger and fries – I hand Michael the Munch print I brought with me. *Anxiety* depicts a group of spectral figures beneath a pulsing red sky, on the same path that features in *The Scream*. "This looks happy," Michael says to my surprise. "Lots of colour, happy and laughter. But a bit lonely. I like it. Who made it?"

Edvard Munch, I tell him.

"Ed?"

"Sure, Ed."

"Maybe Ed will like my words, too." Michael also has a gift for me: a new word, committed to cardboard in his clear and touchingly emphatic handwriting. The word is *disminsh*, which I take to be a play on "diminish". He tells me it means "that the pain vanishes". When I ask, he explains, "You hope it'll be less painful, less discomfort, feeling less bad and horrible. Otherwise the pain is too unbearable, or too deep, all rolled up in blankets." Maybe I could show it to my friends, or to Ed. "Do you think Ed would like it?"

At our fourth and final meeting – 45s, cheeseburger, fries and Fanta orange – I ask if he will ever write another book. He shakes his head determinedly. That publishing gig was too hard on him. "People asked all kinds of questions. Why I did this, why I didn't do that. They were snobby. They made Michael Bernard Loggins nervous and scared. As if I'd done something wrong. Michael Bernard Loggins just did what he had to do." So all there will be in years to come is scattered notes, like the thousands that litter his apartment, written on napkins, envelopes, packets of chicken pot pie. As suddenly as it began, the public phase of Michael's life came to a close. The author of *Fears of Your Life* is too afraid to publish. Even so, he does me the honour of reaching into a garbage bag and offering me a handful of paper scraps covered in his words. "You give gifts, I give gifts," he says. Then he looks me dead in the eye and asks if I will miss Michael Bernard Loggins. I tell him I will and ask if Michael Bernard Loggins will miss Daan Heerma van Voss. He closes his eyes and nods. We say goodbye by not saying goodbye, sidestepping words, nodding in silence.

As I leave his apartment, I still don't know what to make of Michael, how he fits into the story of fear and creativity. Perhaps it is worth returning to Aristotle's explanation of the singular nature of the melancholic in terms of a unique ratio of black bile to the other bodily fluids. Although we have long since ditched the doctrine of the four humours, perhaps there are still lessons to be drawn. The balance between sensitivity and hypersensitivity, between exceptional insight and hallucination, between acute awareness and paranoia, between being spurred on or paralysed by fear, is a balance that is easily upset. Yet for many, it is crucial to the creative process. Melancholy and balance both have their part to play.

Let's start with melancholy, or madness, or fear. What happens when we replace these words with another concept: feeling out of place. A sense of otherness is common to all the artists mentioned in this chapter. It's what gave rise to their need to "tame the world" and go in search of a way to relate to life, a relationship that for them was far from self-evident. It led them to create something that had yet to exist, to express themselves in ways that were original and artistic. Through the centuries, melancholy and fear have prompted millions of self-professed outsiders, unable to express themselves in conventional ways, to paint, write, film or perform in a bid to find meaning in life.

What exactly is an artist? Writer Tim Parks sees them as people who have never found a stable position between the poles of fear and courage, with the result that they are always having to work out where they stand. The origin of their art lies in their response to that instability. Where I belong on the Parks scale is hard to say. But if I had felt at one with the world around me, if I had never found myself wondering why I saw or experienced things differently from my friends, if my imagination had never been captured by something I could not grasp or understand, I would have given up long ago. My notebooks would have remained empty and this book would not have existed. Of this I am sure. In other words, the instability of feeling different and out of place has been both a source of anxiety and a driving force.

This otherness, the inability to find a stable position on the spectrum between fear and courage, says next to nothing about the quality of the artwork produced. That is a romantic cliché, the product of a significant historical bias that has skewed the history of madness and art. Only the greats have been studied to any significant extent: the eminent writers, major poets and world-renowned artists who often cited fear and melancholy as their muses. The poets and artists whose life and work were not lauded by their contemporaries and recorded by biographers have tumbled into oblivion. Never considered worthy of republication or singled out for classic status, their works have to be dredged from obscurity. Yet there is no reason to suppose that these second-tier creatives were any less "crazy" than their celebrated cohorts. I see little point in taking a qualitative approach to madness. Some people who felt themselves to be different produced masterpieces; others wrote down their fears in lists that were mimeographed, stapled and circulated by hand. Some receive global acclaim, others sit at home, afraid that a chicken pot pie might burn away their insides. Some are feted, others withdraw. But when they create, they feel like real people.

It therefore stands to reason that artists can feel an existential loss when their need to tame the world is frustrated. Psychiatrist Jan Swinkels shared with me his experience of treating a young painter, a student at Amsterdam's Rietveld Academy, no older than twenty. He suffered from extreme anxiety and had become psychotic. "Painting was his calling. I prescribed medication, but kept the dose very low. If I gave him too much, he lost the urge to paint, and that was his one way of connecting to the world around him. One of his paintings showed a starry sky and his mother's head in the foreground. He painted a hole in her head and himself standing next to it, holding a shovel." Not long after finishing the painting, the student experienced a very severe psychotic episode. Swinkels was on holiday at the time. "He was admitted to a psychiatric unit and pumped full of drugs. No-one had tried to talk to him. I got a call at my holiday address. He had thrown himself in front of a train." Ivo's parents gave their son's painting to Swinkels. It hangs in his study and he looks at it every day. "I stare at that starry sky, and at the mother's head with the hole in it, and I see a strong similarity. Both the universe and the brain are infinite. You can fall in and never find a place to land. Art is somewhere on that largely uncharted border between biology and psychology, a pure representation of what it is to be human. But that purity comes at a price."

This brings us to balance. Most Romantic poets were aware of what they called their madness, melancholy or anxiety, and could therefore recognise when they were losing touch with reality. They had a certain degree of control, and when they were engulfed by melancholy they usually knew how to find their way out, with a new sheaf of poems as the spoils. Though faint at times, there was always the hope of maintaining some kind of balance. And then there is Michael, who barely has any control over his anxiety. That is why you will never hear Michael waxing lyrical about his fears; he cannot turn them off. For him, it's a matter of sitting them out. His fears lead the way. He follows and keeps score.

My last afternoon in San Francisco is spent walking across the Golden Gate Bridge in the company of former police officer Kevin Briggs. Before meeting up with him, I reread Michael's compendium of fear. No. 138 reads "Fear of Jumping off the Bridge, way up high going down real deep splash in that Deepest water, and then take your own Life away From yourself. You'll Jump from top ledge." The bridge was on Briggs's beat for twenty years, and having read up on its history, he struck me as the man to contact. More than sixteen hundred people have jumped from the bridge since it first opened in 1937. They come from all over the world. Every ten days on average, someone sets foot on the bridge with the intention of never coming back.

We set off on the footpath that runs the length of the bridge, a distance of over one and a half miles. Mist makes a dreamscape of our walk. "I see a different bridge from you," Kevin says. "I see people and wrecked cars. Phantoms no-one would recognise, accidents no one remembers." The traffic thunders past, gusting winds rattle the mesh fences. This is a cold, forbidding place. We wipe our noses and struggle to make ourselves heard. Over the years, Kevin has had to deal with some two hundred people who stood on the edge. Fearful, desperate people, ready to jump. It was up to him to change their minds. Those conversations always came down to fear. Fear of losing face, fear of an uncertain future, fear of letting people down, of not being understood. In Kevin's view, this last fear weighs heavier than most. "People need a way to connect. Either directly or by taking a side route." One of those routes is art. Kevin remembers Jason, a man of thirty-two, calm and polite. "Nothing about him suggested panic or impulsive behaviour. He apologised for what he was about to do. Jason was very smart and sensitive, and incredibly talented, his parents told me later. He wrote books but couldn't get them published. He was different and was given no way to express it. He grew frustrated. Every last hope of connection had turned to pain."

Back home in Amsterdam, I gather the scraps of card and paper Michael gave me and spread them out on my desk. There they lie, alongside a note from D. It dates from long before she left, long before she sent me on this journey. In her hurried, slanting handwriting, it tells me she loves me. That there's no need to be afraid.

# 14

# An Anatomy of Failed Conversations

*(Before she left)*

In the days after my return from San Francisco, memories of
our conversation in the kitchen weave their way back into my
thoughts – the tapping blade on the chopping block, the red of
her sweater. Then come memories from further back. About a
month before she left, she reached a conclusion: my fears had
darkened into depression. I agreed. Perhaps I was relieved that
she had noticed.

This link is not exceptional. "Anxiety underlies depression,"
psychiatrist Witte Hoogendijk believes. "Even if a fear is irrational,
it settles into your thinking, anchors itself in your subconscious."
So it's not so surprising to learn that someone suffering from
depression is three to eight times more likely to have an anxiety
disorder than someone with a clean bill of mental health, while
someone diagnosed with an anxiety disorder is seven to sixty-two
times more likely to experience depression in the subsequent
twelve months than someone without that diagnosis. In many
such cases, depression can be seen as acute systemic exhaustion
resulting from anxiety. British journalist Johann Hari, who has
regularly suffered from depression, compares depression and
anxiety to the same song covered by different bands: a downbeat

emo band versus a screaming heavy metal band. The emotions evoked by the song are very different, but on paper the notes are the same.

How did D. arrive at her conclusion? How did we talk about anxiety and depression? What form did those conversations take? Above all, I remember the question that, with hindsight, has signalled the end of all my relationships: "So what's the matter?"

*

Before the relationship proper, there is being in love. I'm good at being in love. So good in fact that I can even convince myself that this best version of myself is the real me. Whether it's one night only or a passing fancy, a misunderstanding or even an outright mistake on her part or mine, the realisation of how rare, light and liberating such moments are throws me headfirst into the beginnings of love, those weightless first days and weeks when the world seems to keep on expanding, when every detail is infused with meaning and metaphor. I used to think I was an incurable romantic. Now I wonder if I'm just someone who learned early on that it's hard to be in love and depressed at the same time.

Another explanation of my readiness to fall in love is that it allows me to put a positive spin on physical phenomena I usually experience as unsettling. Consider this lyrical love poem by Sappho of Lesbos:

> [. . .] as soon as I glance at you a moment, I
> can't say a thing,
>
> and my tongue stiffens into silence, thin
> flames underneath my skin prickle and spark,
> a rush of blood booms in my ears, and then
> my eyes go dark,

> *and sweat pours coldly over me, and all*
> *my body shakes, suddenly sallower*
> *than summer grass, and death, I fear and feel,*
> *is very near.*

Beautiful, isn't it? An outpouring of love that has also been interpreted as one of the first panic attacks on record.

Twice before D., that feeling of being in love endured. Twice it turned into a relationship: with J. (when I was eighteen) and E. (at twenty-two). J. and E. deserve more than anonymised supporting roles but giving them their due would result in other books and so in this story – on this journey – I will only touch on their response to my anxieties. Though it was never the reason to begin, I soon discovered that being in a relationship soothed my mood. A lover drew me into a world I could easily lose touch with in lonelier times; there were moments of real understanding, of feeling safe from harm. Simon Vestdijk was one of our greatest writers on fear. In addition to fifty-two novels, thirty novellas, around fifteen hundred pages of poetry and numerous essays, he also wrote a dissertation on the subject. As he saw it, love is the primary antidote to fear. Unfortunately for him, he only found love with characters he had dreamed up himself. He told the non-fictional women in his life that he was spoken for.

Another fine example of fear taking a literary route to one-sided love can be found in the work of Marcel Proust. In *Swann's Way*, the first part of *In Search of Lost Time* – his celebrated novel in seven volumes written between 1908 and 1922 – we get to know Marcel as an anxious individual who allows the image of his ideal woman to be overshadowed by maternal fantasies. Just as the young Marcel expected his mother to always be there for him, he expects the same of his great love Albertine. Unfortunately for him, she is an independent being. For Marcel, this is insufferable, unpalatable, inexcusable. It makes him more anxious than he could ever have imagined. The heartbreaking consequence of this love shot through with fear is that Marcel only feels safe with Albertine when she is sleeping, when she cannot turn away or reject him. Vestdijk and Proust: two souls whose longing for connection was so fierce that, ultimately, they chose solitude.

As my own relationships progressed, the question of whether I should share my fears began to hover. It was the right thing to do, wasn't it? Keeping such a secret could only lead to alienation and she was bound to find out one day. But by talking too much, I might overwhelm her. How could I know how many words were enough but not too much, the number that would hold us together?

Earlier I talked about how fear comes in whispers. The precise weight and wording of the whispered message keeps changing, but always amounts to a variant on the same prediction: you're not going to make it. The weight and wording specific to my love life: when she finds out who you really are, she'll be gone in a heartbeat.

And so, in both relationships, with J. and with E., I began to open up. Inching my way through halting, drawn out sentences, I searched for the words to capture my moods and my bad times, my fear of going mad or being seen as a madman. But as I grappled with these formless feelings, the search for words began to take over. As long as I kept talking, there was the promise of a form, of some kind of order. The promise of connection. As soon as I fell silent, I was alone and lost in my own thoughts, wondering if one day I would disappear into them altogether. Once J. and E. had grasped what I was trying to say, I began digging for reassurances. I was going to be alright, wasn't I? We were good together, right? Yes? Do you really mean it? Tell me I'm not going crazy, tell me we can get through this. J. and E. had different – perhaps even diametrically opposed – responses to these confidences.

At my instigation, J. spun a web of reassurances and code words, found ways to soothe and explain. The moments when I asked her how she was doing became less frequent. It was only a matter of time before I had annexed all the words that passed between us and quiet set in. I asked her if she would stay with me.

Without knowing what the question really meant, she said yes. Her expression clouded over. After a while, she began to say things like "But there's really nothing to worry about. Look, the sun is shining." Curtains were flung open, the light roared in. Couldn't I see those trees, the beautiful sky? No, I couldn't. It was like trying to convince someone who is colour-blind of the existence of red.

Loving looks turned pitying, weary, vexed. New words made their way into the bedroom. Medical terms, which she quickly made her own. Words like "disorder" and "depression". Words that had their place, but felt like a condemnation. She was right and I resented it.

E. listened and nodded and then wanted to do fun things together. Go to the movies, eat out, see one stand-up show after another, laugh, get up to mischief and generally muck about. It worked for a while, until I realised the relationship had turned into a distraction.

My fears intruded into both relationships, and my lovers and I had to find ways to respond, without knowing how. Of course, there is never one all-encompassing explanation for why a relationship founders; instead there are dozens, large and small, coexisting and interacting. But in my case, it's a safe bet that one of those reasons was my anxiety and the dynamic it set in motion.

Both relationships reached a terminal phase, where the only reassurance left for me to find was in my lover's tears. As long as she was capable of tears, she still loved me. I began to recognise them; they seemed to follow me.

In both break-ups, the pain was intense, if I'm honest, all-consuming. That sadness had less to do with my lover than with the two of us together. I could not comprehend that something that had once existed and seemed to be everything, was no longer there. When my second relationship ended, I became so confused that, after an episode that a neurologist tentatively labelled an anxiety psychosis, I lost my memory for a day. A phenomenon known as transient global amnesia.

In the months that followed, I put myself back together. I began to come up with explanations for these relational failures. I was too young, not yet ready for love. At other times, a measure of fatalism took hold: perhaps those tears would continue to follow me, perhaps fear would contaminate any attempt at a relationship. Again, I failed to work out whether this was a fear, a portent or a curse. Was I simply better off outside the relationship or, a grimmer prospect, never having a relationship again?

No, that was no way to think.

If love came my way again, it would be different. It would be different and I would be ready.

*

Back to the more recent past and the weeks that led up to D's departure. The apparition my great-grandfather had described as "the old enemy" and my mother had dubbed "the monster" was back to haunt me. It had been skulking around for a while, waiting for its moment.

It was as if, by trying to ignore the early signs, I had passed a tipping point beyond which the situation became exponentially worse. My memory grew weaker, my emotions more unpredictable, my digestive system took on a life of its own and my immune system appeared to be failing on all fronts: I was felled by one virus after another. This undermined me little by little until finally, if only from sheer fatigue, I had no choice but to admit defeat at the hands of an entity about which I knew only one thing for sure: it was stronger than me.

There were still moments of lightness, but these became rarer. They welled up without warning, as I walked down the street or lay in bed with D. batting children's names back and forth, a pleasure we often indulged in. Anything I could come up with was too close to *Star Wars* for her liking. "Boba?" she repeated incredulously. "Solo?!" Her efforts struck me as random sounds rather than names: Per, Falke, Wes, Kit. We laughed – "Right then, no kids for us!" – shrugged and hugged. To this day, I wonder how serious these exchanges were. I beamed when friends saw me with their kids and told me I would make a good dad. At other times, all I could think was: what will I be passing on to them?

Those lighter moments were a blissful relief. See, I can still do it: be happy, make people happy! I craved that relief like a parched man stumbling upon an oasis. He doesn't drink, he guzzles. He doesn't laugh, he cackles. I relished every minute of that happiness, until it ebbed away and its loss made all the things we were missing even more tangible. I tried to explain to her that the monster had relented for a time. She looked at me without understanding.

"So what's the matter?" she asked for the umpteenth time.

Where could I start? I had lost something. It was missing, gone. I had given something away, something that had belonged to the two of us. But what exactly? Nothing. Everything. I didn't know anymore. I knew I shouldn't complain. I didn't want to complain. I complained.

"A trance of supreme discomfort [. . .] trance – I can think of no more apposite word for this state of being." That is how US writer William Styron described his own experience of depression in his book *Darkness Visible* (1990), and that is how it was in the weeks before she left. You sleep as if you are awake and wake as if you are sleeping. You drag yourself from hour to hour. And if that fails, you break down the hours into minutes. You hack away at time until the pieces fit in the palm of your hand.

Mornings were the worst. I would wake up wheezing and shivering, dead tired and anxious. I couldn't make myself eat. What followed was a day in the life of a stowaway or a castaway, a hunter-gatherer whose only preoccupation was to make it through to evening, when my fears would let up slightly. The next day it began again. In search of distraction, I jumped down the rabbit hole of YouTube, stumbled through Tumblr, filled my head with white noise. I watched film after film until they became one endless movie populated by hundreds of actors all talking at cross purposes.

A mantra was what I needed. A magic spell, a sentence I could cling to. I roamed the internet on an endless search for quotes – any guru or charlatan would do, from Buddha to Benny Hill. God, I needed a mantra. I uttered this phrase so often, in my mind and in conversation, that it became a mantra in its own right.

The normal world edged further out of view. In its place was a world inhabited by oblivious millions, people walking around blindly, ordering coffee blindly. A world I could still see, hear and smell, but could no longer touch or feel. The blindingly obvious had become absurdly artificial and, with that, the internal logic that kept the world turning and held it all together had lost its sway. I used to understand that logic and act on it without thinking. I used to be as oblivious as everyone else, but now that was beyond me. These were thoughts I recognised; I'd had them before, during similar periods. Only now they seemed to hold more truth than ever.

I stopped reading books. Words took on a life of their own, derailed sentences, entire paragraphs. On the page, the words "help", "black", "alone" became part of a hidden code. Words like "laughable", "silence", "tired" served the sole purpose of reminding me what a hopeless case I was. Casual connections between things and people had coalesced into a conspiracy. And the plot was all the thicker because I was the only one who could see it.

Everything made noise, nothing made sense. Trucks rumbled through my bedroom, pigeons cooed beneath my pillow. There was a constant pain, dull and diffuse, a kind of pressure exerted on my whole body, clamping down on chest, arms, legs, throat. It was impossible to localise and so could not be fought. All this fed into a fog of self-pity, though it was more than feeling sorry for myself. I felt insignificant rather than pathetic. I saw how vulnerable I was, even if others couldn't see it, or hadn't seen it yet.

I stared at my navel, at my pale face in the mirror, at an altercation on the street corner, at the newspapers, the food banks, the one per cent, the plastic soup, the ozone layer and back at my navel. From big to small and back again. I lent people money knowing I would never get it back. I scrounged dinners off old friends, fathers now, with children whose names I kept forgetting.

Somewhere along the line, "Why me?" morphed into "Why isn't everyone as depressed as I am?" How could people not see what I saw? How could they be so unworldly as not to see all this for the absurd, fragile, desperate circus it was?

I began to look at others the way some parents watch children at play: wistful and a touch envious, dwelling on all the dangers you see and they don't. I felt superior to everyone around me and weaker at the same time. Superior because I could see through their illusions, weaker because I was no longer able to believe and they were. Slowly, I began to resent them for living contentedly, for embracing what looked to me like simple-minded happiness. I grew bitter and self-obsessed. I could hear the condemnations I levelled at myself, but they were no antidote to the bitterness and the obsession. As long as I kept looking for one, I told myself, there was still a road back.

In meek compliance with the myriad rules that shape our daily lives, I brushed my teeth, wiped my arse, stopped at red lights. When I tried to think, my brain groaned into gear, the sentences I uttered were short and feeble. I could feel cognition waning and blankness taking hold. Around mid-morning, I would notice to my own surprise that I had dressed myself, that I was walking down a street, that I was sitting across a table from someone, that I was back in bed.

Someone asked how I was doing.

Yeah, fine. It's all go. You know.

Someone leaned in and said "Cut the crap. What's wrong?"

I forgot what I wanted to say. Words wouldn't come. Lay there on the tip of my dry tongue.

People told me they had tried to call four times the previous day. *How hard is it to pick up the phone?* People told me I didn't call back. *Did you delete my number or what?* A friend whose doorbell I rang told me we had never arranged to meet. Out of pity, he made me a coffee and handed me a biscuit, but he was on his way out and didn't have long. A woman called and asked me why I hadn't turned up. I didn't recognise her voice. She sounded old and forbidding, recriminations thick with spittle.

I contacted my old dealer, who also dealt in "chill pills" – Valium and the like. She said she didn't recognise my number. We talked without listening.

I felt raw, naked, fragile, weary, wasted.

I watched wildlife documentaries and saw myself in sea creatures. The Siamese fighting fish: six centimetres in length, lives in Indonesia's coastal waters and makes himself a nest of froth, a ceiling of bubbles beneath which he and his mate can get cosy. A froth nest struck me as a pinnacle of achievement. How long would the bubbles stay intact? What would it sound like when they burst?

Much of what I saw came in shades of loss. Instead of a street, I saw the trees that had been felled to make way for it. A meatball was a lump of ground-up cow.

My connection to my body changed. At times, I forgot it was there. At other times, it seemed that ownership had been ceded to someone else and I was trapped inside. I stared at the mirror and moved my wooden limbs, a puppet come to life. I knew something was missing. An element had been removed from the vague but barely dissectible continuum of actions, features and traits that constituted "me"; a seemingly insignificant element that was crucial to the balance of the whole. What I saw in the mirror was unreliable, made no sense. Shirt too big, trousers too short.

The bedroom was at once a condemned cell and the centre of my world, perhaps even my universe. The sun rose when I opened the curtains. All was quiet until I hummed, coughed or blurted out some word or other. I became less and less active, could conceive of no movement that would feel better or make more sense than not moving at all.

An overblown podcast on instant noodles sent me off to sleep . . . freeze-dried . . . deep-fried . . . feeding the planet . . . hundreds of billions of packets a year . . . waste . . . the plastic soup . . .

\*

It was all in my head, D. said. And when she said she understood me, I was afraid she was lying, or worse, that she was telling the truth. That truth was even more dangerous; if she understood me now, the time when she no longer did would be harder to stomach.

She comes from a family that has little time for illness. If she came down with flu as a child, her parents sent her to school anyway. Once, when her mother became so ill she had to be hospitalised, she carried on working from the ward, her iPad smuggled between the mint-green sheets. In my case, there were no scans to pinpoint what was wrong; there was no bump, no scrape, no scar. The only evidence came from me: the testimony of someone who appeared to be playing the twin roles of perpetrator and victim.

I talked, she listened. Every time I told her how scared I was I felt relieved, admissions that left me feeling cleansed for a while. She swore to me she didn't think I was lying or exaggerating. But after some urging, she conceded that she believed I was attaching too much value to my feelings, allowing them to carry me away. The word *allow* took a while to process. It implied a choice, the coexistence of two possibilities, either of which might be avoided. So in the end she felt I was taking the wrong option. Nothing was *forcing* me to suffer, after all. She had every right to take that view, but at the time it put a painful distance between us.

Sometimes she told me to try harder. Sometimes she said she wasn't good with weakness. Sometimes she said, "Man up." Words too big to swallow. In all the confusion, had I lost my manhood too? At the end of a day spent chewing over these exchanges, I put this to her. She adamantly denied it. She said I was giving too much weight to words, latching on to formulations. All I could think was: how can you ever understand each other if you don't give weight to words?

She started seeing friends more often. Taking time off from me. That wasn't only in my head.

She asked me why I seemed to come to life in the company of friends or even complete strangers. That was sleight of hand, I explained. A trick that was not entirely a lie, since it drew on inclinations I genuinely possess, and yet it had nothing to do with how I felt, who I was at that moment. Besides, in that kind of company I often felt lonelier than ever. A law of reverse proportionality had come into effect: the larger the group, the more disconnected I felt. Performing that trick, sorely needed at times so as not to alienate people more than was strictly necessary, also left me dead tired. There were pleasant moments too, glimpses of life outside – beyond the depression. But the aftermath of these performances, the domestic transition to my real disposition, that inner collapse, was becoming more arduous. It could take me hours to recover from a conversation that had barely lasted ten minutes.

It was hard to figure out. Was it that I didn't want to be part of the world, to be with others, or was I simply incapable? It was a question I often asked myself, sometimes in wonderment, sometimes in accusation, without hitting upon an answer. As time passed, wanting to and being able to began to mean the same – enviable, hopeful verbs of desire and possibility, two concepts I had lost touch with some time ago and whose existence I was coming to doubt. Until both wanting to and being able to no longer meant anything. I explained these things to her and she looked at me warily. Wasn't it just that I was better off talking to my friends?

No, I said. At most, I might be better off sharing silence with them.

*

A succession of small, painful losses ensued. We had less fun together, stopped going to parties, avoided cafes. It was quiet at the dinner table, we had next to no sex. Sticking at the things we used to enjoy – going to parties anyway, dancing anyway – didn't work either. It only reminded us that life before had been different; different from life during, from life now.

When I went out, I passed from awning to awning, like someone doggedly sheltering from rain. The neighbourhood unravelled in a jumble of numbers and missing street signs. A white façade, the neon-green snake of a pharmacy, stepping into pale fluorescent light. Ibuprofen numbed, though it made my stomach ache. Not so bad, it was a pain I understood: clear, controllable, part of a neat chain of cause and effect, pain with a beginning and an end. On an average income, I calculated, you could buy 21,000 ibuprofen a month. Why this was a comforting thought, I couldn't say, but reasons seemed to matter less and less. My feet were terminally cold and I took to wearing three pairs of socks. Warmth and protection – no harm could befall someone whose feet felt this safe. I bought more socks; they bulged from drawers that no longer closed. On an average income, I calculated, you could buy about four hundred pairs of socks a month.

The strange thing is that at some point, after months and months, this state of total vulnerability, of being turned inside out, feels like your only protection. Because the real terror is not in lying flat out, but in falling. Not rock bottom itself but seconds before, when gravity strikes and you see the stony ground rushing up at you. There you lie. But time passes and rock bottom has its reassurances. You get to know the pebbles, the boulders, the grit. All the pain you feel is familiar. And it starts to dawn that, if things get a little better, if you scrabble to your feet, you can fall all over again.

Not the falling. Anything but that.

"You are a man of leisure, a sleepwalker, a mollusc," French writer Georges Perec wrote in his autobiographical novel *A Man*

*Asleep.* "The definitions vary according to the hour of the day, or the day of the week, but the meaning remains clear enough: you do not really feel cut out for living, for doing, for making; you want only to go on, to go on waiting, and to forget." To wait and to forget, that's what I wanted. I imagined a sleep from which I would wake cheerful and bright. Days of sleep. But why not weeks or months? Or even years?

I read a moving obituary in the newspaper and called a swish restaurant to reserve a table in the name of the dearly departed. An act that gave meaning to my week. It felt like a good thing to do, a pure thing. The idea that someone had saved a place for him gave me comfort. Poor man. Dead. Someone's father, son, husband.

The distance between the life I wanted to live and the one I was living grew day by day. Each day, my life became more unlived. Looking back, I saw a distance I might never bridge again.

Earlier I spoke about the totality of anxiety, the experience of fear and panic striking everywhere at once, felt throughout the body. This totality is temporal as well as physical. When you are engulfed by severe anxiety, you have no sense of how long it will last. If someone were to tell you there's one more day of misery to get through, there might be something to hold on to, perhaps even grip enough for the anxiety to subside. But no-one tells you this, no-one can tell you this, yourself least of all. Ruled by fear, your thinking is corroded to the point where all you can do is ask the question that takes down the last of your defences: "What if this never ends?"

D. felt like she was being dragged into this, dragged under. Was she supposed to let that happen, or let me go? And if we got through this awful time? How long until the next one? Was this to be our life together: a series of quiet, brittle interludes, waiting for the storm to come?

Before long, shameful fantasies of suicide surfaced. I began to concoct all manner of justifications and fallacies. Didn't my inability to lead a normal life mean I had an evolutionary duty to end it, to step aside and make way for those who *were* able, the fittest? Wasn't it woefully self-centred to be such a drain on everyone, to keep inhaling oxygen and ingesting food that was better spent on others? These lines of reasoning became increasingly difficult to refute.

It was all in my head. Objectively, I had – and have – plenty of reasons to want to keep living, and even to love life. I knew this. Of course I did. But the surges of shame at the disconnect between my all-consuming gloom and the objective state of my life – the notion that my feelings were illegitimate, that I was being ungrateful – worked against me and left me feeling guilty as well as miserable. There were kind people who cared about me and this was their reward? All the advantages I'd had in my life caved in on me, became reasons for the world to condemn me, to look at me and say, "You should have been stronger. You should have done better."

Guilt closed in and sent my thoughts racing. Instinctively, I would scan my surroundings for options: a wooden beam, a window that opened all the way, a socket close enough to the shower. These were fantasies, nothing more, and there was nothing romantic about them. They were practical, business-like if anything. People make the mistake of thinking that someone contemplating suicide wants to kill themselves. What they want to kill is something *inside* themselves, the pressure, the sense of confinement, and suicide is the only remedy guaranteed to end all suffering. The one problem being that it destroys everything else in the process. "The person in whom [. . .] invisible agony reaches a certain unendurable level will kill herself the same way a trapped person will eventually jump from the window of a burning high-rise," David Foster Wallace wrote in his novel *Infinite Jest*. "[W]hen the flames get close enough, falling to death becomes the slightly less terrible of two terrors. It's not desiring the fall; it's terror of the flames."

Fantasies like these used to panic me but, for a few years now, I have seen them as hopeful: they are a sign that I want to escape at all costs, which suggests that I want to live at all costs. Back then, I had yet to find this hope, which has helped me to a point where these fantasies seldom trouble me. At most, they live on as a twinge of acknowledgement and compassion when I hear of someone who has committed suicide, as if they were hit by a bullet that narrowly missed me.

*

The anatomy of another failed conversation:

> Me: Can you tell me again that it will be alright?
> Her: It'll be alright.
> Me: Can you say "Don't be afraid?"
> Her: You don't have to be afraid.
> Me: I don't?
> Her: I hate that you feel this way.
> Me: But?
> Her: But can't you . . .? No, never mind.
> Me: What?
> Her: Nothing.
> Me: Tell me.
> Her: Can't you try to get over it?
> Me: What do you think I'm trying to do?
> Her: Can't you try a little harder?
> Me: You think I'm putting this on.
> Her: No. But we're good together. We are, aren't we?
> Me: It's not you. Honestly, not at all. I love you. What if I can't get my work back on track?
> Her: Work's not the be-all and end-all, is it?
> Me: Would you say that if I was destitute?
> Her: I can't help thinking: if you were really happy with me, you wouldn't feel this way.
> Me: This is something I've always had.
> Her: Then maybe you haven't found the one. The other

day, when your friends came over, it was like there was nothing wrong. You were cheerful, you were funny.

Me: I was pretending. I can only keep it up for so long and it leaves me shattered.

Her: Can't you pretend more often?

Me: I don't want to pretend, not with you.

Her: It would help.

Me: I love you. I love you so much.

Her: You're only saying that because you need me now.

Me: It's what I feel. I'm not sure of much, but I am sure of that.

Her: Tell me you love me when you're feeling better. When it counts again.

Me: You think I'm putting all this on.

Her: No, I just think that you sometimes get bogged down in it.

Me: I really wish you could feel what it's like, to be in my shoes for a while.

Her: That's a horrible thing to say.

Me: Not out of spite. Just so you could see it and feel it for yourself. So we could talk about the same thing.

Her: So what *are* we talking about?

[SILENCE]

Me: Can you tell me again that it will be alright?

Her: It'll be alright.

EXIT "Her". "Me" stays put for a while: cranky, tired. Trying to work out exactly where the conversation went off the rails. As if that would make a difference.

\*

Talking in circles, variations on the same conversation, hundreds of them. And when you've had that conversation a hundred times, why not a hundred and one? Over and over.

The more she reassured me, the more I came to depend on it and the more emphatic the next reassurance had to be. After a while, it wore her down. The words ran out. But I felt compelled to go on explaining. This was such an essential part of me, I had to make her understand how I felt. If she understood, we could move on, start again.

She didn't think it would be that easy. She had begun to see me as someone else. Even my voice was different, reedy and out of whack. In a way, she was right. A human being amounts to little more than the sum of their traits. And many of my better qualities had turned bad: loyalty had withered into dependence, imagination twisted into a source of paranoia. Trying to explain that this "someone else" was my shadow, my navigator, and that one day he would fade into the background again was no use. And I needed her so badly. Separation anxiety had never really been part of my make-up, but at that time I couldn't bear to be without her. Fear of separation? Yes, but at its core it was the feeling that I wouldn't make it, the fear of going under. The more I think about it, the more I realise that at that time it was less about love and more about survival for me. And in her own way, she had set her sights on survival too: throwing herself into every aspect of her life that she could control – her job as a journalist, her exercise classes, her nutrition plan – a regime as impressive as it was oppressive. Her life went on, only it consisted of more and more control and less and less of me.

Playwright Sarah Kane characterised the hope of a depressed person seeking support from loved ones in her final play *4.48 Psychosis*, one of the finest accounts of the inner world of depression I know: "I came to you hoping to be healed. You are my doctor, my saviour, my omnipotent judge, my priest, my god, the surgeon of my soul. And I am your proselyte to sanity." Kane knew exactly what she was doing when she mixed the medical (doctor, surgeon), the religious (omnipotent, saviour, god, proselyte) and the legal (judge): underlining the all-important nature of contact with the other, every conversation charged with the urgency of one last chance. William Styron describes how, during his depression, his wife became "nanny, mommy, comforter, priestess and, most important, confidante. . ."

I could see that D. was toying with the thought of leaving me. I responded with every outpouring of love she had once wanted to hear. Why could I only declare love now that I was in danger of losing it? I didn't know the answer. All I knew was that she couldn't just abandon me. "You abandon a child," she corrected me. "You leave an adult."

*

Before our conversation in the kitchen, she had gone to the market with a friend. She told her friend about my behaviour and asked if it was normal. The friend shook her head and asked why she was still with me. She'd had to think for a moment and her silence, the absence of an answer, came as a shock to her. She told me this as we talked in the kitchen. The memory comes to me suddenly, as if I hadn't really heard her at the time. "Don't be afraid," I remember saying. "It'll be alright." Words that sounded awkward coming from my mouth, like I was speaking someone else's lines. She sighed and asked what she was supposed to tell our future children when I felt this way. *Daddy isn't feeling well?* And what if I passed this on to them? (Far from unlikely, given the links between anxiety and heredity.) No, she wasn't going to say that to her children. She refused. What kind of life would that be?

"You mean for little Boba and little Solo?" I ventured.

She shook her head.

She left.

# 15

## *Talking in Colours*
### *(After she left)*

She left and the process of inner decay slowed and then stopped. With no-one around me, I began to stand on my own two feet, little by little, day by day. By taking the journey she had handed to me, by reading endlessly, by attending clinics and conferences and getting to know fellow fearties, I gradually found myself on steadier ground.

From my many conversations, I learned that there is a dichotomy between people who have experienced an episode of depression or severe anxiety and those who have not. From the perspective of fear, the former are the insiders, the latter the outsiders. The gulf between one and the other, they told me, is almost impossible to bridge with words; the very thing I had tried so many times to achieve.

One reason why this is so hard to do is because the experience of depression or severe anxiety cannot be expressed by cataloguing the physical and emotional symptoms. Listlessness, overstimulation, anxiety, the need to make your world ever safer and ever smaller: we know these vignettes by now. But to share in the feeling of being stranded in that dark, claustrophobic world on the other side, in what it's like to go on living when all you want to do is withdraw from life? This is all but impossible unless you have been there.

In our attempts to explain, we insiders resort to imagery, comparisons with objects or phenomena that are more widely known: it's like being under water or at the bottom of a deep well, like you can't breathe, like drifting, like drowning, like ageing decades in days. "I feel like I'm eighty years old," says the unnamed protagonist in Sarah Kane's *4.48 Psychosis*. "I'm tired of my life and my mind wants to die." A dissenting voice says, "That's a metaphor, not reality." The protagonist gets the last word: "It's not a metaphor, it's a simile, but even if it were true, the defining feature of a metaphor is that it's real." That last puzzling sentence is nonetheless recognisable: sometimes a metaphor or a simile is the only meaningful linguistic vehicle for sharing your experience, your reality.

The work of systems biologist Denis Noble, Professor Emeritus at Oxford, led me to Wittgenstein's metaphor of the ladder to understanding. Climb a ladder, and when you reach the top, everything feels logical and self-evident. It's a wonderful vantage point to have. You can oversee everything, understanding is yours. Not only that, but you can throw away the ladder; why would you ever want to go back down it again? All well and good, but you needed the ladder to get you there in the first place.

*

There is a long tradition of representing illness through metaphors (Susan Sontag's *Illness as Metaphor* is a great place to start, if you are interested). Many of these comparisons are militaristic in tone: battling bravely against cancer, Covid as the invisible enemy. To recover from illness is to emerge victorious. And of course these metaphors have their cruel side, implying that those who "lose the battle" should have done more, fought harder. Insult is added to injury: those ravaged by illness are expected to shoulder the blame.

So much for illness in general. It is in describing mental health problems, so much harder to grasp than purely physical ailments, that the metaphor really comes into its own, with a rich variety of images that are often exuberant or even poetic. Depression or anxiety is a dog chasing you, an all-enveloping fog or a life lived under glass. The metaphors vary from one insider to another, and even from day to day, but with a number of common denominators: they speak of oppression, a barrier to human connection, no way out.

Roughly speaking, depression-anxiety metaphors can be grouped into four main categories. The *descent*: into the ravine, the catacombs, the pit. (There's a good reason why people talk about feeling down.) The *jailer*: I feel trapped, paralysed, desperate to escape. The *hollow*: a deep sense of emptiness. And then there is *darkness*: a black cloud, murky water.

While insisting that our state of being defies comparison, so many of us turn to the same images in our despair. We could bemoan our lack of originality in doing so, but for me there is a comfort and a beauty in this. Even when we are at our most lost and alone, our words tell us we are still connected.

\*

## METAPHORS OF FEAR, COURTESY OF MY FELLOW FEARTIES

A circle you can't get out of.
*Anita*

A slippery mountain you have to climb.
*Elisa*

It was like I was stuck in a heavy,
indigestible, sickening pea soup.
*Minka*

A coat that's way too tight.
*Eva*

Like being attached to a rubber band that keeps
pulling me back, like walking into a glass wall, like
being on an endless roller coaster, like wandering
around at the bottom of a pitch-black pit.
*Anita Brigitta*

A whirlpool.
*Corinne*

An abyss.
*Mirjam H.*

A beast inside of you that sleeps and wakes up, and the
more attention you feed it the stronger it becomes.
*Wesley*

Never-ending rain.
*Thea*

A stressed-out watchdog.
*Mirjam D.*

A chain around my leg that keeps pulling me down.
*Manon*

A bucket I keep falling into.
*Hans*

A monster that took my life from me three years ago.
*Marion*

A storm of compulsive thoughts.
*Desirée*

A lie you believe. Sometimes a flash of
lightning, sometimes a smouldering fire.
*Daaf*

Fear is like a car coming straight at you and
you can't stop it, and you can't step aside either,
and you're probably wearing the wrong kind of
shoes, and so you fall. You're always falling.
*Michael Bernard Loggins*

\*

Few writers say more about the link between metaphor, anxiety and depression than Sylvia Plath, and not only in her poetry
and her celebrated novel *The Bell Jar*. In 2015, linguistics expert
Zsófia Demjén used cutting-edge analysis software to study Plath's
writing. The poet's journals proved to be a particularly valuable
source for anyone interested in the language of the insider. One
of Demjén's key findings was that Plath used significantly more
metaphors to describe a negative state of mind than a neutral or
more positive state. Findings such as these have led scholars to
view density of metaphor as a linguistic indicator of emotional
intensity. Plath's negative metaphors were also wilder, more lyrical and more intense than her positive ones. Demjén sees this as
evidence that Plath experienced negative emotions more deeply
than positive emotions, but I would offer a different explanation:
that the need to find the right words to express a negative state of
mind was a matter of life or death for Plath at her loneliest and
most misunderstood. Finding the right words for a more positive
state of mind was more of a writerly exercise.

Plath favours the jailer metaphor for depression: no less than
28 per cent of the metaphors in her journals can be grouped
under that heading. Some examples: ". . . to see his mind [that of
friend Dick Norton] soaring, reaching, and mine caged." Or: "Stop

thinking selfishly of razors & self-wounds & going out and ending it all. Your room is not your prison. You are." Another metaphor to which Plath frequently returned is that of emptiness, the hollow vessel. This passage speaks volumes: "I am afraid. I am not solid, but hollow. I feel behind my eyes a numb, paralyzed cavern, a pit of hell, a mimicking nothingness. I never thought, I never wrote, I never suffered. I want to kill myself, to escape from responsibility, to crawl back abjectly into the womb. I do not know who I am, where I am going . . ."

Another aspect of Plath's language in more troubled times is her use of absolutes: "always" or "never", "everything" or "nothing", "everyone" or "no-one", as opposed to the more nuanced wording she used to interpret life when she was feeling better. This is part of a wider phenomenon. In 2018, the journal *Clinical Psychological Science* published an extensive scientific study showing that the language of people experiencing depression differs fundamentally from that of people on the other side of that line. So much so that scientists even claim they can tell whether someone is depressed based on the language they use.

Someone with depression is far more likely to use the first person singular (I, me) and much less likely to use the second or third person singular (you, he or she): their gaze is turned inward and they are less attentive to others, less engaged with the world around them. Psychologist and data scientist Johannes Eichstaedt of the University of Pennsylvania calls this "I Language". The main conclusion of his wide-ranging 2018 study of Facebook accounts is that Facebook users who struggle with their mental health use I Language relatively frequently. They have an above-average preoccupation with how they feel, while Facebookers without these issues are more likely to post about politics or family, topics that demonstrate an interest in the world. Eichstaedt gives "tears", "crying", "pain", "miss", "hate" and "ugh" as examples of other words that may indicate depression. He believes it is only a matter of time before we have algorithms capable of predicting which Facebook users will go on to develop depression.

Plath's journals show a similar pattern: the worse things get for her, the more words she reserves for herself. At times, she even addresses the depressed part of herself directly, in the "you" form. "An outlet you need, and they are sealed. You live night and day in the dark, cramped prison you have made for yourself."

Night and day, in the dark, imprisoned.

Describing her inner struggle, she says she is "afraid that the disease which eats away at the pith of my body with merciless impersonality will break forth in obvious sores and warts. . ." Her journals are not a place of muted sadness but of constant conflict, a civil war between the part of herself that wanted to live and the part that could not bear to. It was a high-stakes battle for control. The means was language, and nothing else.

As Plath's depression grew more life-threatening, her journal entries became sparser, more pared down. On 6 July 1953, she told herself "First think: here is your room – here is your life, your mind: don't panic. Begin writing, even if it is only rough & ununified [. . .] If you can't think outside yourself, you can't write."

"What I fear most," she wrote, ". . . is the death of the imagination."

Later, in *The Bell Jar*, she would write "The silence depressed me. It wasn't the silence of silence. It was my own silence."

It is as if Plath could no longer reach her words. A few weeks after 6 July 1953, she attempted suicide. Almost ten years later she would turn on the gas oven and try again.

*

Since D. left, there have been no more panic attacks. I find myself checking my phone less often. Only rarely do I catch myself wondering what I will say when I see her again. Two months have passed and the longer she is gone, the more I see how right she was. I was using the wrong words. Insisting this could *never* end well. Asking why she *always* had to react like that. Why *no-one* understood how *hopeless* it all seemed. Speaking in absolutes, I twisted reality into a zero-sum game.

Reading and talking have helped me along. Research and writing help too. I have found precedents and explanations, even for the most inexplicable of my thoughts, including the hidden codes I convinced myself I was seeing and hearing. These were delusions, relational delusions to be precise, faulty rearrangements of logic that mess with the laws of cause and effect. Things that had nothing to do with each other suddenly appeared to be related while self-evident connections fell apart, so that everything seemed to be charged with a deeper meaning that was being withheld from me. German psychiatrist and philosopher Viktor von Gebsattel called this the *Gegenwelt* – a counter-world of the imagination into which anxious people can disappear. The counter-world resembles the world as it was before anxiety took hold, but only outwardly. Instead it is governed by malicious whispers, unsettling pacts and disturbing thoughts that refuse to be tamed. In almost all cases, I am relieved to read, the phenomenon disappears by itself, merging back into reality so gradually that you would be hard-pressed to say where the counter-world ends and the normal world resumes.

In short, the fragments are rearranging themselves and starting to point in roughly the same direction once more. Perhaps even her direction, I sometimes allow myself to think.

\*

And then, one nondescript day at the end of the second month, D. calls me out of the blue. Her voice is soft, quiet, starved of oxygen. She suggests taking a different tack, a middle ground between two homes. Spending part of the week with me, the rest at her friend's place. A holding pattern, only for a while, until she comes back for good.

Her words trigger an overwhelming emotion, part love, part weariness, but I can't find anything to say. The emotion quickly drains away, too quickly. This is not what I had hoped for.

"But then," I say at last, as if struck by a revelation, "it will be like you're leaving, over and over."

"No," she answers, "I'll be coming back again and again."

We are quiet for a while.

Wasn't that always the plan? she says. To see where we stood after a while?

Yes, of course it was.

Don't I miss her?

I do. A lot.

So why can't she come back? She accuses me of stubbornness and pride, traits I possess in abundance, but which I don't think are playing much of a part in my response. After a strange, guerrilla-like exchange full of diversionary tactics and sudden outbursts, a peaceful silence settles in.

When we have nothing more to say, I am the one who hangs up.

*

Before I can give myself over to a relationship again, to that ambiguous, fragile covenant, I need to see myself through her eyes. What did she see when she looked at me? What did she smell? What did she hear?

She saw someone whose appearance changed. Whose lips became chapped. When I was on my meds, I piled on weight. Not that this happened all by itself. It was hard work, involving muffins, gingerbread, anything I could stuff my face with. And when I tried to stop, I lost so much weight she called me skinny.

She saw someone who at times was capable of making an intelligent, urbane impression in the public eye. Someone who, only days before her departure, had sat in front of an audience at a Swedish book fair and – cool as you like – held forth on the dire state of Dutch democracy but who, as soon as the performance was over and we were alone again, dashed back to our hotel room, slid under the covers and would only move to grab the remote so as not to miss a minute of the Kavanaugh hearings, which he endured while foaming at the mouth about the world going to hell in a handcart, thereby demonstrating that the depressive is a visionary rather than a madman. She was not impressed.

She smelled someone who sweated profusely. A pile of whiffy shirts in the laundry basket, the sum total of a single hot day. She smelled sourness on my breath. Metallic. Chemical. She heard teeth chatter. A voice that was pinched and childlike, not the voice she knew as mine. But perhaps worst of all, I had ruined birds.

The phrase comes from another insider, actor and writer Todd Hanson, once quoted as saying "if you're not at least a little bit depressed, you're just not fucking paying attention." Hanson was telling a friend about a conversation he'd had while out walking one day. On the way, his walking companion had made a concerted effort to lighten the mood. "Look at the positive things in the world. Listen to the birds in the trees. Can you hear the birds in the trees? The birds are singing. Listen to the birds singing."

To which Todd replied, "I appreciate what you're trying to do, but when I hear those birds singing, I'm not hearing the happy twittering of happy little creatures. I'm hearing the screams of ter-ritorial animals that are either competing for mates or competing for some sort of feeding territory against other competitors which will starve them out if they don't win, and in the kill-or-be-killed, eat-or-be-eaten cauldron of murder that constitutes the natural world, that's what I hear when I hear the birds in the trees."

The friend he was telling all this to said, "Yeah, but you were in a really bad space at that time so you were hallucinating, you were hearing something that wasn't there . . ."

"Well, I was definitely in a depressed state," Todd agreed, "but I wasn't hearing sounds that weren't there. I was hearing the real sounds of the birds."

"But you were wrong because when birds sing they're happy," the friend said.

"Well, technically they're singing because of territorial—"

And before Todd could finish, his friend jumped in and said, "Todd. Don't ruin birds for me."

I had ruined birds for D. I had pointed at the trees and dismissed them as worthless. I was a colour-blind man trying to convince her there was no such thing as colour.

My thumbs begin to tap my phone screen. They put together a text, a message that says I'd really like to see her again. She answers quickly – dinner, the day after tomorrow.

I yank open the wardrobe. What to wear, what to wear? Shirt or sweater, jeans or chinos. The day after tomorrow.

What could she and I have done differently? We could have tried to understand each other's language. It didn't help when I listed symptoms, physical symptoms, and then treated her like a doctor. Nor did it help when I resorted to overly complicated metaphors, which invited qualifications like "far-fetched" and "over the top". What really didn't help, in my case, was thinking back to when it had all seemed so natural. Sometimes I noticed that she was holding me up to the light of the past for inspection; her memories had become implicit promises of what life was going to be like, of the strong, dependable man I would turn out to be. I knew I wasn't who I had been. I was failing the inspection and began to hate it. We could have built a new system of meaning. An Esperanto for Unfortunates. There could have been two insiders, not just one.

To my mind, the colour spectrum would form a good basis for that Esperanto. Ever since we humans obtained evolutionary benefits from distinguishing one colour from the next, colour recognition has worked pretty much the same for all of us. Which is why there are such strong similarities in the feelings colours evoke across various cultures. Red speaks of energy, action, power; grey is dull and ominous; green is positive and hopeful. Around the world, in all age groups, white prompts positive associations and black tends towards negative. A black mood. Black as night. Black humour. A black hole. Black represents the mysterious, the hidden, the unknown. In evolutionary terms, humans have always depended on sight for survival, and depended on light to see. To see black, a harbinger of death, all we have to do is close our eyes.

Through centuries of painting, black has symbolised death, depression or weariness of life. For modern examples, we need only think of Kazimir Malevich's *Black Square* (1915), an all-black canvas that changed painting for ever. This was not a depiction of a black object, it was not pictorial; it represented a state of mind. As Jackson Pollock grew older and his battles with alcoholism and depression became grimmer, colour disappeared from his work. From 1951, it barely featured at all. Mark Rothko's *The Black Paintings* consist mostly of black and grey blocks separated by a thin white line. It was Rothko's last series. Separated from his wife and suffering from depression, in February 1970 he took an overdose and severed an artery in his right arm.

In 2010, scientists at the University of Freiburg conducted a study involving retina scans and demonstrated how colour literally disappears from the lives of people with depression. Our eyes are designed to transmit every possible colour nuance to the brain, but depression puts a dampener on this process; a type of colour correction occurs, as if a matt filter has been placed over the visual input. As depression deepens, lead researcher Dr Ludger Tebartz van Elst explains, the cells at the backs of our eyes convert less light into nerve signals and as a result our brains perceive less colour. This also dims the contrast with which we see the world. People enmeshed in major mental health problems look out at an ashen grey landscape. Lack of dopamine is the culprit: this neurotransmitter is key to how the cells at the back of our eyes function but in the throes of depression, it is in very short supply.

Some of the insiders I have spoken to talk about their state of mind in terms of colour. Black is a hopeless day; yellow is problematic; red indicates clarity and energy; blue denotes relative calm.

This saves them trotting out a list of symptoms and sidesteps the tendency to assign blame. They and their loved ones or caregivers can jointly decide that this is a black day and either leave well alone or attempt to lighten the shade a little. To quote Stephen Fry: "Try to understand the blackness, lethargy, hopelessness, and loneliness they're going through. Be there for them when they come through the other side. It's hard to be a friend to someone who's depressed, but it is one of the kindest, noblest, and best things you will ever do."

It seems like an age since I last saw D. But I needed that time, I tell myself. Little by little, thanks to the people I have met and the things I have seen and read, I have regained something of myself. Perhaps I should be grateful to her for leaving.

Shirt. Chinos. Day after tomorrow.

*

I walk through the door to be greeted by a white dot of a nose and long black whiskers: a cat's features on a child's face, looking up at me. We stare at each other for a moment. It's as if I have stepped into a dream with eyes wide open. I nod and Cat Boy lets me pass.

As I look around the restaurant from our regular table by the fountain, the scene retains its dreamlike mood. I feel detached, floating between memory and sensation. The thought of her sitting across from me again in fifteen minutes' time feels unreal, like a rumour I've chosen to believe, without knowing why. The reservation is in her name and the scrawl on the paper tablecloth is missing its exclamation mark. Laura, our favourite waitress, stops by and asks me if we have something to celebrate. "I haven't seen you in such a while, I thought this must be a special occasion. I have an instinct for that kind of thing."

As soon as her back is turned, I slather an oven-warmed roll in butter and ram it in my cakehole. Then I send D. a text to say that a boy disguised as a cat is stealing our bread.

*See you in ten*, she texts back. *Running late.*

The minutes drag by, sweaty, breathless, dislocated.

My pocket begins to vibrate. It's Pepijn. His voice is distorted, coughing, sucking in air: he's in the middle of a panic attack. We breathe together, deep inhalations, slow exhalations. When he is calm enough, he asks me if it's going to be alright.

"Not a hope," I reply.

Relieved laughter fizzes down the line. We promise to call each other tomorrow. "I'm waiting for my date," I say.

"Shit! That was tonight. Of course! Just tell her you're her ticket in the lottery of life."

"I'm not sure that's—"

"Not the winning ticket. But a ticket nonetheless."

As soon as I hang up, I see her. She holds out her arms. We kiss full on the lips, a hug, an embrace. It all comes rushing back. The sweetness of the perfume I know so well but couldn't begin to describe, the necklace I gave her for her birthday. Not everything is familiar. Her sweater is new, white with horizontal blue stripes. Just your style, I tell her.

"And what's that exactly?"

"Nautical chic? A jaunty old sea dog making a go of it at Harvard."

She laughs. I made her laugh again.

"I'm sorry I ruined birds," I say.

"What's that supposed to mean?"

"I just wanted to say I'm sorry."

"Then say it."

"I'm sorry."

"Yeah, well, we're just going have to get better at this. The break has been good for us, and now we can move on. Sorry is a bore." She puts one hand on mine and brushes a crumb from the corner of my mouth with the other. A crinkle appears at the corner of her left eye, lines I've never noticed before. She has changed but I have too, I note after a few swallows of Beaujolais.

You could say I've spent all my adult life clinging to the belief that romantic love would fix me. A belief that set two unconscious and unstoppable processes in motion. First, every time my love – any kind of love – slipped away into the depressing twilight zone that clued-in friends called "a relationship crisis", I would cling to the object of my affections. Even if I didn't really want to stay with her, I just couldn't let it be over. Second, this belief that love would fix me implied that I was deeply flawed, perhaps even broken. And so every love perpetuated the cycle: as long as there was someone who had to fix me, I was still broken. Perhaps for the first time in my life, the pattern has revealed itself to me, a pattern I need to renounce as soon as possible, if not for my own sake, then for my lover's.

We order. Salads, fish, wine. More wine.

Her use of the word "we" in connection with the future gives me enough confidence to ask what she's been up to lately. As soon as I say it out loud, it feels like we really are on a date. A date is a promise. I promise not to lean on her again. She promises not to be my fixer. I went to the gym, she says. I worked hard. Early nights and a healthy diet. It sounds like an elaborate purification ritual, and why shouldn't it be? "You look well on it," I say, a touch too fast, as if someone is whispering prompts in my ear.

"What about you?" she asks. "Did you take that journey I suggested?"

"Yes, I did." All those faces – from Jaap Kunst to Batman, from Marina to Japie, from my fellow fearties to the young striker in his pink CR7 boots, from Pepijn to Michael. All those stories. "The harbour's in sight and you wouldn't believe where this old tub has taken us," I say, giving her my best Captain Birdseye.

"Us?" she asks with a hint of jealousy.

We eat, talk, drink, laugh, talk, eat, and drink some more. I consider asking her about the tears she shed in our kitchen, where they went, if they are still around. But that would be sentimental, unnecessary, inauthentic. We order our standard dessert. A ginger cake, which we solemnly swear to split down the middle. A promise I break by claiming the bigger half.

When we step outside, I see that she has secured her bicycle to mine. So this is how the journey ends, I say to myself. With this soft-focus image of loving attachment. The love I always hoped for and wanted to believe in.

I fool myself all over again.

# 16

## *Mother of Dragons*

The sound of church bells fades on the salt air as I step onto the platform. I have travelled west to the North Sea coast to meet two men who found themselves in a crisis similar to my own but did not get back on their feet, whose lives buckled under the weight of their fears. Walking from the station, I pass a string of cheery signs: Chin Chin, a nightclub; Chef Amigo, a fast food place; Amazing Asia, the local Chinese takeaway. The world according to the seaside town of Zandvoort.

This is not an epilogue, I tell myself. Our love still exists, it goes on. I love D. as much as ever, perhaps more than ever – feelings amplified by my relief at her coming back. Yes, she came back. That evening, months ago, we unlocked our bikes outside the restaurant and she cycled back to my place, to our place. She returned the next day with the rest of her things. It was all I could do not to burst into applause as she came up the stairs with her bags. An unadulterated happy ending to this story, one I had hoped for all along. It has proved to be an illusion.

Something has altered since her return, something that is hard to express but impossible to ignore, however much I've tried. She lies beside me again, snuggles up to me when she is cold. Those lingering looks are back, her eyes seem the same. And yet. Now that she is back, I keep leaving the house. I keep leaving. One morning, during a silent breakfast, I find myself wondering: what if the journey doesn't end at the final destination but continues until the changes it has wrought have played themselves out in the minds of the travellers. As much as I wanted everything to stay the same, I was still changing.

It's not that I resent her leaving. I respect her decision, it was something she needed to do. Perhaps it's that her journey has been very different to mine. After a meandering detour, through my family's past, through science and literature, through history and philosophy, I have begun feeling my way towards a new language that might save us. Her journey was clearer, more linear: the leg that put distance between her and my fears, and the leg back. "I love you as much as I hate your fears," she said one Saturday after-noon as we sat in the living room. Down the street, someone had wheeled out a barrel organ to pep up the shoppers. As it tootled away, I struggled to dissect her thinking and was left with a notion of her love and her hate in a balance that hovered around zero. "I think you're wonderful," she continued. "But suddenly there's this intruder, this fear, and it changes you. It makes me think that I'm not enough. That the life we have isn't enough for you."

It wasn't her fault, it wasn't our fault. But there was no way of explaining this to her. And because I was in a better place than I had been when she left, and because I loved her, I accepted that this was how she felt. It was the only way to stay together.

Continuing along the promenade, a tepid drizzle sets in and I quicken my stride. Hurried steps, as if someone is hot on my heels.

Getting back together was not an easy ride. Our words tore into each other on a regular basis. I told her I was struggling to feel safe with her and she took this as a reproach. On mornings when I felt anxious, she didn't believe me when I said I loved her. It didn't help that these are words that don't come easily to me on a daily basis. She was convinced I only said them when I needed her. I blinked and felt the tears: six years together and still I couldn't show her the difference between love and panic.

"Tears won't help," she said. "Trying harder might."

"You mean trying harder to pretend?"

"Sometimes trying harder and pretending amount to the same thing."

I sided with love and worked to keep the intruder at bay. I banned him from our life. I resolved not ask her for reassurance again and kept my fears to myself, where no-one could find them.

In a way, it worked. In the weeks and months that followed, I asked no-one for reassurance, for love, for support. I did it on my own. But when friends observed that I seemed unusually quiet these days, a little low, it was hard to deny. The life D. and I led, the good life, the enviable life, began to feel more and more like a facsimile. She said she was pleased with how things were going, told mutual friends that our break had done us good, that we were better than ever. Very occasionally, I tried to say that I still found it difficult to feel secure. What did it mean that she had felt the need to leave, what did that say about our future?

It didn't say that much, she thought. Besides, things were good between us, better than ever.

My insecurities remained. She didn't feel the need to keep talking about them. It was up to me to flip the switch and trust her again.

I wanted that. It had to happen, I would find a way. "Where is that switch?"

"It's a metaphorical switch."

"How do you find a metaphorical switch?"

She shook her head.

In the heart of Zandvoort, on a street tucked well away from the beach, he is at the door to meet me. The door to what officialdom calls a "sheltered living facility": a small block of flats where round-the-clock care is available for people whose mental state makes it impossible for them to live independently, overwhelmed by the fear and confusion they experience on a daily basis. The man at the door, a member of the care team, is Japie. That's right, the boy who christened me "Lard Arse" on a football pitch all those years ago.

One way to process the unexpected alienation that had come with D.'s return was to hammer away at a punch bag on a daily basis. Some days it was easier to believe I was Batman than others. I walked into the boxing school one morning to find him standing there in the middle of the mat: Japie. A tiger up his left arm, a black panther down his right. In the locker room, I worked up the courage to speak to him. The first thing he did was correct me: it was Jaap, not Japie these days. He recognised me from years gone by. Just as I was about to go back there myself and remind him how he had belittled me as a kid, he mentioned that he worked in the mental health sector. I asked him how anxiety impacted his patients and he said he had a tale or two to tell. We agreed to meet at a cafe a week later.

It had all started with an ad for the Salvation Army, looking for counsellors to help troubled youngsters. Jaap wound up working there for years, topping up the salary he earned four days a week with two nights as a bouncer. From there, he became a probation officer. "I saw every disorder going: psychoses, schizophrenia, split personality, borderline." His next job was as a paramedic driver for the ambulance service. "As an ex-bouncer, I knew how to handle myself and I wasn't fazed by a splash of blood." When he'd had enough of the ambulance life, someone advised him to get into social work, a career move that led to the facility in Zandvoort. In the course of a single conversation, Japie my football club nemesis had grown into Jaap, a man I could only admire for his choices and the role he played in the lives of others. On so many levels, he was living a more generous, more courageous life than my own. Courage that went far beyond the written word.

I asked him about the people he helped and Jaap sketched lives warped by fear. "When they feel like a failure, they say they're not themselves." By "themselves", he explained, they meant their ideal self: the person who should be holding down a steady job, living in a home of their own, with a partner and a couple of kids. "They don't realise that person is a figment of their imagination. We're not talking about people who read books and are into self-analysis. Many of them stay on their feet by *not* thinking things through." Though fragile, they found a way of life that worked for them, clinging to a fixed daily routine and drugs that may or may not be helping. And as they lived that life, contact with others became increasingly strained and harder to handle. They smoked, ate too much or far too little. Their skin turned pasty, their teeth went bad. The trickle of correspondence dried up and eventually leaving the house became too much for them. The longer they stayed indoors the more frightening life outdoors became, the life all those other people were blithely leading, as if there were nothing to it.

Jaap welcomes me to his workplace with a firm boxer's handshake. An assortment of autumn leaves have scurried into the foyer behind me. The cramped bodies of two dead bees on the windowsill catch my eye as I register the flatulent smell of overcooked cauliflower and a central heating system on overdrive. This is home to Jack and Terry (not their real names), who have agreed to talk to me about their anxiety. About what it means to live a life scarred by chronic fear.

They are ready and waiting for me in a sweltering third-floor common room. Jack is fifty. Terry tells me he was born in 1976 and tries to work out his age from there but comes unstuck in time. A regular occurrence, Jaap explains. On the five-point severity index that health insurers use to gauge their care quotient, Jack is a three and Terry a four. That's health care labels for you: why use a name when you can use a number? The personal experiences of insiders are clustered into symptoms, practical criteria for determining health or illness and for identifying "chronic cases" like the two men in front of me. The power of the system is legitimised by objectivist, scientific language, by classifications, taxonomies and scales. But pick apart the statistics, reach the core and you find yourself talking to real people, to Jack and Terry.

Terry and Jack are both depressed and anxious, although Jack is on the mend. For years he was terrified of becoming homeless. He lived with his mother, who suffered from dementia, and was plagued by worries about the future. Belligerence became a way to master his fears. He got into a fight with the neighbours, who were always banging on about his hedge. The police got involved. "I couldn't keep a lid on things anymore. It all got out of hand, and I ended up here."

Terry still has psychotic episodes during which he does all kinds of things that he can't recall later. Does he really forget everything? "Not everything," Terry says. "The one thing hardwired into my brain is that I have to feed the cat. Even if I stay indoors for months and don't see anyone, even if I neglect myself, I never forget the cat. That's just not on." I picture a bewildered phantom wandering through a darkened flat in search of a tin of Whiskas.

Jaap explains that Terry's woes have been compounded by people's attempts to help him. Terry's family are Thai and view his mental fragility as a demonic form of weakness. His sister once treated him with rose petals to drive away the evil spirits thought to be dwelling within him. When that didn't work, he was dragged to a temple for an exorcism: a ritual associated with the Mesopotamians, the first people to recognise what we now call depression. They used exorcism to revive the spirits of overly lethargic citizens. And of course it is associated with medieval Europeans, whose view of mental illness as satanic led to thousands of death sentences and failed attempts to drive out the devil. But the devil would not leave Terry and he came to be blamed for all the family's misfortunes, from financial setbacks to the death of his grandmother six years before our meeting. This made Terry more anxious than ever. In the meantime, he has made peace with his grandmother. He tells me he still sees her regularly. She comes and sits by his bed. She doesn't say much, but her presence feels peaceful. Her first appearances sent Terry into a panic, but nowadays he enjoys her company.

Jack doesn't have an easy relationship with his family either. "They think I should find myself a job. Like them, like everybody else in the world. They see me as a sad case."

Are Terry and Jack on medication?

Jack is on Aripiprazole, an antipsychotic.

Terry isn't on meds. "When I take them, it's like everything is happening in slow motion. All they do is make me sluggish. I don't want to be like that. That's not me."

Do they want to go back to living independently one day?

Terry doesn't. "I'll end up losing my way again. I've stopped thinking about the future. Getting through the day is hard enough."

Jack does want independence: a job and a girlfriend, the sooner the better. He is eager, impatient, to get his life back on track.

Out of nowhere, Jack asks how I met Jaap. I hesitate, but after everything I've heard, I don't want to lie, not to them. So I tell them about that day at football practice, about Jaap's "Lard Arse" quip. Much to my own surprise, I make it sound like an amusing anecdote I've told a hundred times before. Jaap can't remember a thing about it. He goes to say something, but stops. Terry fills the silence with what I should have said: that we're all just getting along as best we can.

Two weeks later, I visit Jack and Terry again. Jack remembers me, Terry draws a blank. Even so, he trusts me enough to show me a series of pictures he has painted: nine portraits of fairy-tale beauties with flowing tresses. Based on photographs of models and actresses, these are portraits of fantasies rather than real people. "The guys in the common room tell me I painted them, but I can't remember." He offers to give me one. I say I couldn't possibly accept. "Why not? It's not like I made them. Not really. Please." There is a pleading edge to his voice, as if the paintings are not just an outlet but also a burden, a reminder that he is not like most artists. I choose a portrait of Daenerys Stormborn of House Targaryen, a protagonist of *Game of Thrones*, destined to rule the Seven Kingdoms with three dragons at her beck and call. Once she takes the throne, she wants to rule justly and halt the cycle of violence. She wants to break the wheel.

Half an hour later I'm back on the train to Amsterdam, with Terry's Daenerys for company. As the dunes give way to the flat green fields of northern Holland, it dawns on me that, all things considered, life could be a good deal worse for Jack and Terry. They live relatively stable lives, can call for help at any time, and have Jaap and each other to talk to. Meanwhile, others teeter on the brink or slip through the safety net society has put in place. People so lonely that they not only have thoughts of suicide, but are prepared to act on them. The hopeless, the desperate, the almost lost. In the end, what sets them apart from me and you, those of us who live more or less normal lives? To put it in the starkest, most heartless of terms, where does crazy end and healthy begin? When people pose a risk to themselves and others, when they experience a crushing inability to be happy, when they repeatedly sabotage their own lives and the lives of others, we can speak of pathological behaviour, or perhaps even an illness. (Which raises the question of how we then deal with that illness.) But what about the vast majority of people handed the label of an anxiety disorder? Are they all actually ill?

Months ago, when I began this book, I considered myself lucky to be living in an age when, for the first time in history, we have a real sense of what anxiety is; a situation analogous to that of a hospital patient after Ignaz Semmelweis's scientific breakthroughs on antiseptic procedures were finally put into practice. In light of what I have learned since, that starting point strikes me as hope-lessly naive.

I spend the trip mulling over my own experiences of anxiety and how they are echoed in a multitude of testimonies and scientific works. As the train pulls into my hometown, it strikes me that the dividing line between normal levels of anxiety and pathological anxiety is far more problematic than I initially thought. Not because the symptoms associated with extreme anxiety – panic, alienation, the terrifying prospect of losing your mind – are not serious; they most certainly are. But because susceptibility to anxiety turns out to be distributed remarkably evenly across the world's population, comparably to other characteristics, such as height or intelligence. It follows the pattern of normal distribution. Time to piss off the maths-averse schoolboy I once was and liven things up with a graph.

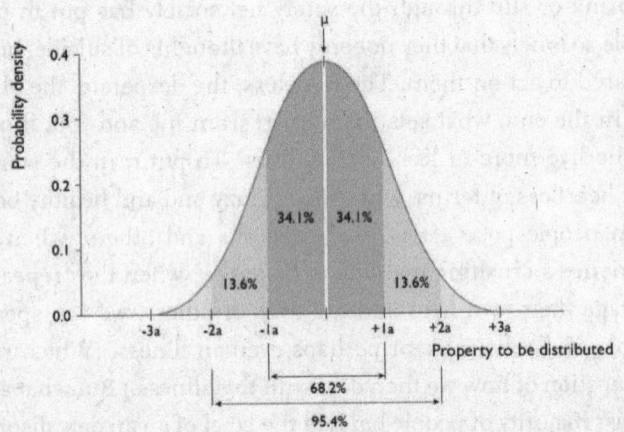

Regardless of time and place, within each population there is a large middle group of 68.2 per cent which converges around the mean (within one standard deviation). Then there is a smaller group of 27.2 per cent that is further dispersed from the mean (two standard deviations), either positively (e.g. by being taller/

more intelligent/more anxious) or negatively (by being less so). The remaining 4.6 per cent is made up of the extreme cases at either end of the spectrum (three standard deviations). Within a group, there is always a subset of people with exceptionally high levels of a particular trait, and a subset of people with very low levels of that trait. This leads me to ask a question with major implications for how we view society: how meaningful is it to put the 31.8 per cent of people outside the large middle group in a separate category, and give them a separate label?

Take height for example, an excess of which is associated with all kinds of health issues. What would happen if we came up with the special label "giant" to refer to people who are exceptionally tall? Two mechanisms would come into play: those within the "normal" spread would start to see the giants as strange exceptions, and the giants would come to view themselves as abnormal. Our fixation on categories and taxonomies has led to a major misconception regarding exceptional cases: the notion that they represent a distinct group that is fundamentally different from the rest of us. In reality, the exceptions – those who officially suffer from a disorder – are at a point a little further from the mean, nothing more. This has led many neuroscientists to champion neurodiversity, the idea that the brain has so many variations that affect our mental functions (learning ability, sociability, moods) that it makes far more sense to view these variations not as abnormalities, but as degrees of difference across a broad spectrum.

It is worth noting that these degrees of difference probably have some evolutionary benefit, otherwise they would have been eliminated by natural selection. A condition such as haemochromatosis, for example, which causes the body to retain excessive levels of iron, has been linked to resistance to tuberculosis. Scientists have also speculated that higher glucose levels in the blood due to diabetes may have offered our ancestors protection from freezing temperatures; without this abnormal mutation, in other words, it is possible that large groups of people in northern and western

Europe would not have survived the Ice Age. From an evolutionary perspective, the people we have just labelled giants would have been valuable members of a hunter-gatherer community, especially well suited to protecting the tribe. A similar claim can be made for above-average anxiety: just as a group needs bravehearts and daredevils, it also benefits from people with a heightened awareness of drawbacks, imminent disaster or impending doom. Without fear and people who tend towards anxiety, the human race would have been toast a long time ago. In short, anxiety is a common and often useful trait, not the preserve of a bunch of misfits. It is a trait we all possess to some degree.

We need only step back in time to appreciate how relative the labels we use for excessive anxiety really are: an imbalance of the humours (Hippocrates); intemperance (the Stoics); melancholy (the Romantics); neurasthenia or nervous debility (the time of my great-grandfather Jaap Kunst); depression (my grandmother's time); phallic narcissism or neuroticism (my mother's time); and finally, anxiety disorder (my own day and age). The simple fact that being born in another time can mean living in a completely different psychological-medical reality should leave us feeling at least a little humble as to what we know or think we know. Not that I am out to equate the theory of the four humours with the insights of modern science; it is hardly going out on a limb to acknowledge that we know more about all kinds of mental health problems than we ever did before. But at the same time, that overwhelming body of knowledge, symbolised by and manifested in the DSM, has brought about a fundamental shift in our idea of health. According to the DSM and the doctors who rely on it – and, by extension, most of society – mental health has come to mean the absence of negative symptoms, a life without side effects. But in my view, health is concerned with how we function, how we feel when we get up in the morning and go to sleep at night, our degree of dependence on remedies and the care of others. Health is not an absence, but the presence of vitality and resilience, qualities you can hone by proving to yourself and others that you can handle situations despite feelings of anxiety, not by seeking to dispel them at all costs.

The more we see anxiety as a collective issue, the greater the solidarity we show. The modern history of anxiety (dating roughly from the birth of the anxiety disorder in 1980) has been a history of exclusion. I am not talking about physical exclusion; most people with heightened anxiety manage to steer clear of a facility or a clinic unless their fears erupt into violence or psychosis. The exclusion I am talking about is both subtler and more widespread: a mental exclusion of labels and categories accompanied by all manner of medication. Like Pepijn, people with heightened anxiety can all too easily end up in a pharmacological pinball machine, saddled with the idea that they may never fully become part of the community, that there is something fundamentally wrong with them, something they need to suppress or excise. But, more than anything else, they are vulnerable, and the sad truth is that vulnerability often leads to sorrow, pain and struggle, to setbacks and crises. By treating anxiety as something we all experience to a greater or lesser degree – a trait that has played a part in our evolution as a species – we invite discussion, reflection and acceptance. To regard it as a disorder is to say that there is something wrong with those who have it, that they are ill and need professional help – but not necessarily our help.

My scepticism about disorders may seem strange in light of earlier reflections. I remember all too well the relief I felt at having the label "anxiety disorder" conferred on me, and I know from experience how much accepting (or even embracing) such a label can mean to someone who doubts the legitimacy of their symptoms. But that enlightening benefit, I realise, is worth less to me now that I understand the many disadvantages associated with thinking in terms of labels and disorders.

First, there is the damage it does to your self-esteem. To say you are vulnerable to anxieties is to accept that this sensitivity is an intrinsic part of who you are; it's an attitude that can lead to self-examination, that enables you to know yourself better. To say you have an anxiety disorder is to run the risk of conflating your personality with that label, a position that all too easily encourages you to swap self-examination for medication under the cover of an officially sanctioned illness. And as you take the tablets and learn, as a patient, to identify with the one part of yourself that stands in the way of you becoming a fully functioning human being, you often start to think less of yourself and to withdraw unnecessarily, because (often without realising it) you have started to see yourself as the victim of a parasitic disorder that stands between you and your real self. Recent research at the University of Groningen shows that the degree to which you maintain your autonomy (i.e. do not "hand it over" to a label) affects the persistence of anxiety symptoms; people with a strong internal locus of control, who believe they can influence the course of their life, are less likely to have a chronic anxiety disorder than those with a strong external locus of control. Autonomy pays.

Another drawback of labels is that, once attributed, they can undermine our much-needed willingness to show solidarity. In 1997, Professor Sheila Mehta of Auburn University in the US state of Alabama conducted an interesting study which looked at whether characterising a person's state of mind as an illness causes people to act more or less kindly towards them. The experiment began with a group of people gathered in a room on the pretext that they would be participating in an experiment on learning behaviour. While they waited, an actor posing as one of the subjects struck up a conversation and told another subject that he was suffering from a mental health problem. In one group he described his problem in terms of his biochemistry (genes), while in the other group he put it down to things that had happened to him (life events). The actor then went into an adjacent room and the subjects were told that the test centred on his learning behaviour. His task was to press a bunch of buttons in a certain order and, if he made a mistake, the subjects were to administer a mild electric shock. (No shock was actually administered; the actor feigned his responses). The findings revealed that participants who believed that the man's illness was due to his biochemical state administered more shocks than those who believed he was the victim of life events. Professor Mehta's study suggests that believing a disorder to be rooted in objective, biological causes does not make us kinder to the vulnerable; if anything, it appears to make us harsher. Today, as the impact of Covid on our mental health is becoming clearer, solidarity and empathy are two qualities we need more than ever.

Every time someone uses the term disorder, it's worth asking what they mean. Would imbalance be a better description? Could pattern be preferable to symptom? Instead of focusing on a cure, might we look at ways of adapting? Could we use the word "trait" as an alternative to "illness"? Could a diagnosis be characterised as "a cluster of behavioural traits"? In proposing these alternatives, I do not want to suggest for one moment that the issues people are struggling with are any less serious. But this is not simply a matter of wordplay: the language we use can change our idea of what someone is going through and ultimately change how we look at the person themselves.

A plea for vulnerability? Yes, I believe that is a plea worth making, although in today's media landscape we need to keep a watchful eye out for the tendency to overcompensate or even glorify our vulnerable side. Let me explain.

Thankfully, the idea that the taboo on anxiety disorders (and other forms of mental illness) needs to be lifted is gaining wider acceptance. But there are some serious drawbacks to the well-meaning way we go about this. It follows a set format: a well-known individual goes public and talks about the problems they have overcome. While this openness helps lift the taboo, it can also start a vicious circle: the media zoom in on the "frayed psyche" of the person in their sights and that person then feels the need to live up to this image in order to hold the public's interest.

I found myself being part of this culture for a while. Under the banner of open-heartedness and transparency, I sometimes talked about my fears in interviews in the hope that I would feel liberated if I didn't pretend to be stronger than I was. I talked about the "chemicals in my brain" that caused my fears, a choice of words that not only elevated me above others without these exceptional chemicals but also absolved me from further self-examination. The unsavoury part of all this was not talking about personal problems; I still believe in the legitimacy and necessity of talking or writing about these things. No, it was the misguided notion that this made me somehow special or even unique.

The testimonies of psychologically troubled public figures are valuable in terms of raising public awareness and tolerance but there is a catch, in the shape of an implicit silver lining. The reader or viewer knows from the outset that a celebrity's mental health issues have not caused them irreparable damage. They are still worthy of media attention, after all, which suggests that they are lauded, rich, enviable. Those who fall permanently by the wayside are rarely if ever interviewed. It is also worth remembering that, however full and frank they may seem, celebrity testimonies are always censored to some degree: revelations are aired as long as the experience can be romanticised or hint at hidden depths in the teller's public persona. Otherwise, what's in it for them? In many ways, it's a modern-day twist on the Romantic obsession with melancholy.

This trend has spawned a subcategory of academic analysis known as celebrity studies, which focuses on the specific mores of celebrities and their influence on popular culture. In recent years, many articles in the field have been devoted to the "celebrity meltdown": the mental collapse of someone in the public eye, often accompanied by spectacular drug and alcohol abuse. This "train wreck" usually takes place in the full glare of public scrutiny and, following an intervention, the person in question goes on to give candid interviews about what is then rebranded as a "dark time in their life". The celebrity meltdown is almost always couched in terms of an inability to cope with the rigours of success, a portrayal that conveniently feeds back into a popular culture obsessed with fame and fortune. A prime example of this mechanism is the career of singer and former child star Demi Lovato, who struggles with eating disorders, bipolar disorder and anxiety. In 2013, she published the bestseller *Staying Strong*, a book in which she shares her day-by-day insights about life. *Stay* is tattooed on her left wrist, *strong* on her right. Encouraging words that do no harm. One year after *Staying Strong*, she went on to launch a new cosmetics range with the tagline *skin care is self-care*, a commercial exercise in equating spiritual self-sufficiency with purchasing and using cosmetics. In other words, the woman who told us to stay strong is now appealing to the insecure narcissist in us.

I am not out to claim that these testimonies are disingenuous, or that Lovato's suffering was not genuine. Intimate accounts of personal struggle can be sincere and honest, even while they are being converted into cold hard cash. But their sincerity and honesty doesn't stop them being problematic. Perhaps this is best expressed by fellow fearty Corinne, one of the people I met at the ADF conference on anxiety: "When a big DJ [. . .] or a chat show host or a vlogger talks about how depression or anxiety gets in their way, I often think: yes, but it's only natural for them to fall apart sometimes. They lead hectic lives, everyone wants a piece of them. I'm just a simple soul with a boring life. And yet here I am with anxiety. What reason do I have? And that makes me feel angrier and more frustrated with myself."

I have serious reservations about presenting psychological problems as something precious that brings you a fuller and richer experience of life than the average, less troubled person, about calling it a silent force, as some overly optimistic therapists have done. It is tempting to believe in this kind of poetic justice, in a feat of linguistic dexterity like Jeanette Winterson's eloquent phrase "the nearness of the wound to the gift". Or the words of Natalie Diaz, in her beautiful poem "From the Desire Field":

> Let me call my anxiety, desire, then.
> Let me call it, a garden.
> [. . .]
> because when the shade of night comes,
> I am a field of it, of any worry ready to flower in my chest.
>
> My mind in the dark is una bestia, unfocused,
> hot.

A wonderful, lyrical description of how wildly fear can thrash around when your hold on reality is at its weakest (in the dark), and the disturbing beauty in letting your panic sprawl and seethe. But for me, Diaz's observation towards the poem's conclusion feels more genuine:

> And even though you said today you felt better,
> and it is so late in this poem, is it okay to be clear
> to say, I don't feel good [. . .]

I can't help feeling that most of us who don't feel good haven't the faintest idea how to go about calling our anxiety desire. How would that work? What good would it do us? Singing to your tormentor after the fact – once the fear has subsided – is not without value, but it is a relative value that shouldn't lull us into a false sense of security. Almost all of the fearties I have spoken to, from Michael Bernard Loggins to Jack and Terry, would be only too happy to shake free of their excessive fears. *Desire? A silent force?* Why should everything exist to empower us? Why pin our hopes on that one limited benefit making us a more successful person, a worthier parent, a better employee? If we are so eager to rebrand our vulnerabilities as strengths, are we really taking them seriously? If the only way to endure our slumps and our lows is by turning them into stepping stones, chapters in the story of future success, aren't we simply paving the way to collapse all over again?

Pondering this balancing act – the challenge of acknowledging fear as a shared trait that holds some benefits without glorifying the vulnerability at its heart – I leave the train and walk through Amsterdam Central, the station that has been the starting point of every leg of my journey to date.

As this book nears its conclusion, it may create the illusion that both my journey and my fears are at an end, that I have somehow conquered or even defeated them. But the truth is that, for many of us, the fears go on. I will never lose that vulnerability, no matter how much I want to. Things will be fine for a while, I will feel happy and that happiness will feel natural. Then it will start to feel less natural, and then it will disappear. The old enemy will stir, the monster. But happiness will come again. Come and go, come and go. I will have to accept the waves as they roll in. With the passing of the years, I hope that the highs and lows will even out a little but the underlying swell will never completely disappear. I no longer believe in healing, because I no longer fully believe in the illness. And I choose to see that as a position of hope. The tables of the station bookshop are stacked with self-help books. But self-help is a contradiction in terms. Help will always involve others: writers, therapists, loved ones, friends. We need others and they need us in return.

I head home with Daenerys Stormborn tucked under my arm. D. stares in wonder at the painting and declares it the ugliest thing she has ever seen. I smile. It's a thing alright and yes, it's ugly as fuck. I take the Mother of Dragons to my study and slide her in among my admin folders, where she stays for weeks. During that time, I tidy the room. I order my notes, pack my well-thumbed books on anxiety into boxes and stow some of them away in the attic.

One evening, D. asks if I've thrown "the thing" away yet.

I shake my head.

Why not?

It will be months before I can answer that question. By then we will be on holiday, in a place far away.

# 17

## Breaking the Wheel

We are lying on a bed in an Airbnb basement flat on the other side of the Atlantic. Two weeks off. Today was spent tramping along the coastline. We pressed our palms to the trunks of giant redwood trees and ate omelettes at a hilltop diner, staring silently at the ocean. As we lie dozing, the owner's dogs yap in the courtyard. The vague scent of hashish lingers; our landlord likes to light a pipe and watch vintage horror movies deep into the night.

When the silence lasts too long, she tells me she loves me. I love her too, more than I have ever loved anyone. I say the words, but they fail to convince. My legs won't stop shaking. We went out for dinner in Berkeley and I spent the twenty minutes waiting on the subway home pacing up and down the platform. It put her on edge, she asked what was wrong. I said I didn't know. Trains raced past, no clue where from or where to.

To be honest, I have been restless for months. The panic has dimmed in recent weeks, but I have less and less to say. My book, my journey, remains unfinished and I can't shake the frustration. Something is keeping me from working up my notes into a final chapter without feeling like a charlatan. Lying on this bed, I realise it all has to do with what she once called the intruder.

\*

In hindsight, I have been able to piece together what was going on. The fears that bring so much misery are also deeply connected to who I am, to my thoughts, my way of thinking about and experiencing life. The intruder is part of me. By maintaining that some parts of me had a right to exist (and were even worth loving) while other parts had to disappear, I was gradually pulling myself apart. I was doing what Jaap's problem cases so often do: confusing my ideal self with my real self. And in that confusion, I had split myself in two. Maintaining that kind of division eats away at your energy and the strain becomes hard to hide. Living up to the facsimile of our life together was leaving me numb. It occurred to me that I could hire an actor who bore a reasonable resemblance to play my part and it might make her a good deal happier than she had been with me. If she noticed the difference at all.

It wasn't as if all the love and enjoyment had disappeared from our lives. We took a spur-of-the-moment holiday, tore around an island on a scooter, her arms wrapped around me, her cheek pressed against my neck. When she cooked, I would sneak into the kitchen and steal a mouthful from the pan when she wasn't looking, only to have her chase me away with a ladle, Punch-and-Judy style. There was still evidence enough for our love, reason enough to believe in a future. Yet it seemed to me that she had developed a full-blown allergy to the least suggestion of fear or worry, a struggle she dared not admit because she still loved me and wanted so much for this to work. And so the struggle was never played out as a struggle, but as an insoluble internal contradiction. This ushered in a silence. It left a chill.

I had begun knocking back a few glasses of whisky of an evening; the first time in my life that I craved alcohol. I made more time for friends who rolled the best joints, and insisted they leave me a supply. At the party we threw to celebrate both our birthdays, I took LSD (and by all accounts was cheerful as could be). In short, it was taking increasing amounts of poison for me to pretend to be someone else. My body began to feel the strain. Hers played up too, an uncomfortable ache in her jaw, especially after difficult conversations. But our home was no longer a place of consolation. Caught in a dynamic we could not put into words, we were slowly turning into extreme versions of ourselves; she grew harsher, I withdrew. Both of us became quieter and more ruthless. We sought protection in limiting our exposure to each other. A good day was one I had trouble remembering the next.

One night, I woke up bathed in sweat. At first, we concluded that this wasn't all that unusual for me. Then came a raw, ugly rasp of a cough. I asked D. if I should be worried, a question I had asked hundreds of times in all kinds of ways, and so her automatic response was matter-of-fact. People get coughs, she said. It happens. A few days later, my phlegm was flecked with blood and I asked my question again. Nothing out of the ordinary, she said, just a ruptured blood vessel in my throat. She is not a doctor but she talks with the firmness of a doctor, a tone that sounds like it's backed by facts, scans and studies. I used to love that firmness.

A few days passed and my hold on reality began to slip. One night I was convinced that I could feel time leaving scratches on my face. A little while later I was convinced that I was D., that I was inside her body looking out at myself. Her hands were my hands; I stretched, sniffed my wrists and inhaled her perfume. Morning came. I tried to match words to this experience and concluded that I must be delirious. D., who was dressing for work, thought this was impossible because I hadn't said anything for at least half an hour. I took my temperature: 41 degrees. Should I be worried? She didn't think so. Fever was only a danger to infants and small children.

But what if I had pneumonia?

"Daan, this isn't a Russian play. Nobody gets pneumonia nowadays." She weighed her words and thought she might have been too hard on me. "If you want to be sure, call the doctor." She pressed a kiss to my hot, damp forehead and went to work. "See you tonight." Footsteps died away and off in the distance a front door closed. Echoing silence, a ringing in my ears. I called and the doctor instructed me to come as soon as I could. I staggered down the stairs and found a cab. I was diagnosed with pneumonia and prescribed a hefty regimen of antibiotics.

Lying beside her that night, I felt that I had disappointed her. Or worse, that she had come to despise me and the weakness of my body. Whether or not the pneumonia has something to do with the rift inside me, she was not to blame. Any more than she was to blame for the substances I was taking to achieve a state of numbness.

The whole notion of blame is irrelevant. As I see it now, she was doing what she could. I thought that I was doing what I could. No, that wasn't quite true. To a degree, I had let in the separation between us. After a string of attempts to have a conversation, I ended up clinging to my own wounds, rather than the small chance of reconciliation that might still exist.

When the fever had gone, I packed my suitcase and went travelling, to places I had already been. My stated aim was to finish this book, but it felt more like following in my own footsteps, trying to track myself down. On my way back, I would find myself planning my next trip. I told myself I was someone who liked leaving. This was a lie. I had become someone less eager to come home.

I would return to a dark house. She knew what time I would be back and that it unsettled me to find the place empty. But after every trip, I returned to find her gone – out with friends, out alone. I didn't blame her, but it was hard not to read it as a sign. When we were at home together, I felt a muted nostalgia for another time, when we could say we loved each other without a trace of pain in our voices. I had begun writing letters: to friends, and to a woman I had met, someone who asked me questions that forced me to think purely and honestly about myself. In my incipient correspondence with her, I felt a freedom I hadn't known in a while. It made me curious but at the same time left me feeling dejected: what exactly did this say about my love for D.? Whatever it said, this was not an epilogue, I told myself. In no way was this an epilogue.

I said it felt like I was on a dead-end street. Another step each day, never looking forward.

You are not on a dead-end street, she replied in a customer-service tone.

"Tell me you love me," she said one night. She sounded beaten, as if she was giving in to something, requesting a lullaby that had once meant the world to her. I obeyed and the words didn't work, they spoke only of obedience.

A winter came and went. I stopped saying I loved her because I was afraid she would reject it. Once she said, "I think you want to end this, but you're waiting for me to make the move. Well, I'm not going to."

Here we are, lying on a bed in a basement flat on the other side of the Atlantic. Dogs are yapping and the last whiff of hash fades from the air. She tells me she loves me. I say the words back at her. As she snuggles up to me, I whisper that I'm not going to be able to do this anymore. Our last conversation as lovers has begun.

As I whisper, I touch my face. My skin is hot but tight, as if a film has been stretched over it. I don't feel fear anymore. I don't feel anything. And then Daenerys Stormborn appears in my mind: the dragon mother, the wheel breaker, the fantasy portrait gathering dust in my room. It's an ugly thing alright, but is that all there is to say about it? Isn't there beauty in someone like Terry – disowned by his family, fiercely loyal to his cat – pouring his feelings into a creative act, though he knows that later he will remember nothing about it? You can call it strange, abnormal, even a show of weakness. But I don't want to. I refuse. This book has no ending because I haven't absorbed the thoughts and ideas I have come across in writing it. I advocate acceptance, but still see my own fear as an intruder. I advocate profound, sincere changes in how we treat each other while I live out a facsimile. I have spoken to dozens of people without listening to myself. I ask for their honesty, while I dissemble.

Setting out on this journey, I characterised fear as my navigator, refusing to share the road map. As time went on, I came to see him as a shapeshifter. Fear is wired into our genetic make-up, but it is so much more than that. Fear can spawn panic or lead to withdrawal from the world; it can be channelled into aggression or creativity. Fear is an illness, but never quite the same one. This explains the zigzag route I have taken. To home in on one of those manifestations would have run counter to what I see as the essential characteristic of anxiety: its multiplicity. And I felt I could only do it justice by taking different approaches and perspectives, by shifting between reporter, fellow fearty, historian, journalist and writer. But now, on this holiday, at the end of the ride, I understand that I've got the metaphor all wrong: fear is not the other, neither intruder nor navigator. Fear is in the workings of the car itself, part of the machine. For some of us fear is engine and chassis in one, for others no more than a gear they seldom use. But fear is part of us, and part of me.

There is no way to love me and hate my fears. They are part of me, part of my character, and even intrinsic to some of the better aspects of who I am; a certain sensitivity, the importance I place on empathy, the attention I give to what I try to do, the gratitude I can feel for everyday happiness. Lying on this bed, I think of Jung's image of the shadow and feel sure that unless I try to integrate my shadow side into who I am, and soon, I will start to fall apart. The holes inside will grow, swallow parts of me that I will never be able to find again. And once that happens, I will be beyond the help of love, the poet's remedy for anxiety. These things slot into place as I lie here beside D., the woman I love, the one who sent me on this journey, a journey that was supposed to lead me to insights that could save our relationship. Neither of us could have suspected, thought, or even feared that it would lead not to a rebirth but to an ending. That the insight gained would go beyond what we had intended and lead to a clear sense that things would never work out between us.

She doesn't respond. Perhaps my sentence was too much of a whisper.

I say the words again, louder this time. The trembling in my legs stops.

She detaches herself from me and asks what I mean.

Everything, I say. Us. I can't do it anymore.

It feels like I'm talking to myself, but she understands every word. Ten days or ten years? A question from long ago and the answer no longer matters. Both points on the horizon feel equally distant.

She asks me again if I really love her.

Of course, I do. Of course.

Bullshit, she says.

No, it's not.

Why tell me this now? she asks. Why here? In the middle of a holiday we've been looking forward to so much?

I tell her again that I can't go on. And why here? It dawns on me much later that I wouldn't have been able to say the words back home. At home, they would have felt like a betrayal of every shelf and drawer, every wall we had painted, every flower she had bought at the corner stall. Here, on this holiday, on this bed, there is only the two of us to hurt.

She tells me not to hide behind the word "can't". When it's wanting to that matters. Wanting to be together. Finding a way to flip the switch.

Again. I can't *do* this anymore.

Her face tightens. She wants me to take more responsibility for what comes next. She wants me to say the words, as if to break some kind of spell.

I can't see any other way, I say. Then, step by step, I waver my way from *I can't do this anymore* to the colder assertion of *It's over*.

It is as if she needs those words to propel her into motion, an acceleration that can only be understood by accepting that this conversation and this farewell have been coming for some time. Her determination to keep us together turns at a single stroke into a determination to separate us as quickly as possible. She grabs her phone and starts Googling fares and flights.

She asks if I know that our home will no longer exist when I return. Her voice is calm and steady, as if describing a law of nature.

Still unable to gauge the deeper implications of this knowledge, I tell her I do. Any other answer could only invite accusations of cowardice.

You don't need to leave like this, I say.

She wonders what point there could be in staying.

I don't have an answer ready. We could talk, I venture. Give ourselves some closure? Hug a few redwoods, look at the ocean together?

She shakes her head.

Within thirty minutes, her ticket is rebooked. Her flight leaves in a matter of hours. No point wasting more words on this. Our lexicon is tainted, old intimacies sullied, reassurances dry enough to choke on.

We try to catch a little sleep. I take the couch, she curls up on the double bed.

Somewhere in those lost, dark hours between night and morning I climb into bed beside her. I want to see the sweet curve of her back, breathe her in. Perhaps it will all be less real, less final, if I lie with her. Her warm neck, the downy hairs on her earlobes, have become matters for observation; I am a witness, no longer a participant. My lips brush her shoulder; she wakes with a jolt and pushes me away. My teeth start to chatter. She shoos me back to the couch. So, I think to myself, these are the events of our last night together.

Pale morning light floods our basement.

At half past five she says she's sorry she doesn't know how

my book will end. I tell her she does, a comment she chooses to ignore. I never imagined that my journey, this book, would end this way; because I started out not knowing what I would find, and because I never thought for a second that our love would end like this. She starts to pack. I get in the way, like an old man unsure of his bearings. She jettisons the guidebooks she handpicked for our trip and tosses me the shirt she sometimes sleeps in – it's back to being mine.

On the basement doorstep, we hold each other for a long time, but she already feels different, colder. She wishes me all the best in life, I wish her the same. I stand there in my underpants, shivering, teeth chattering, and wave her off. She turns twice and waves like she has hundreds of times. Like she will never wave at me again.

I hear the rattle of her suitcase wheels, muffled snatches of her conversation with the Uber driver, then silence. It will be six weeks before I hear her voice again. Over the phone, she tells me she's doing well, that she feels strong. We talk for a while, it's hard to say what about. She takes a deep breath and says: I am stronger than you. I have always been stronger.

As I return to the basement, the owner's dogs come pattering down the stairs and gaze up at me without barking. I look around the flat and, seeing she has left me the toothpaste, I start to cry. Though the words on my screen quiver and jump, I write her a long, loving letter to which she will never reply.

Hours later, pale and weary, I am strolling around a resort that has become a ghost town. But there is more than just misery. An energy wells up inside me, a force I don't particularly want to feel, that doesn't seem appropriate. What was once whole is now broken. What is broken might now begin to heal.

I pick up my pace. Bright sunlight, sharp shadows. I send a message to the handful of friends we have in common and ask them to take care of her, to be as good to her as I once tried to be. Then I drop Pepijn a line. I say I hope he is doing well and that we should arrange to meet up when I get home. He responds immediately, miraculously. His fears seem to be subsiding, he writes. And life isn't bad at all. I can almost taste the disbelief in his words. I smile and turn off my phone.

Strangely enough, I don't feel anxious. Even the anxiety that comes with finishing this book, with completing the journey, maintains a respectful distance. Though there is plenty left to fear.

I know that the kitchen where this journey, this book, once began will soon no longer exist. It will be broken down into its constituent parts: the oven, the knives, the breadbox. She will take with her what was ours, and is now hers again.

I know that she will take all kinds of things, but she will leave Daenerys Targaryen. The wheel breaker and I are condemned to each other.

And I know that I will stop taking my medication. Not today, not tomorrow, but one day soon. It's time to bid the system farewell. I cannot stop the DSM regime from turning, but I can remove a single spoke, myself, from the wheel. Eventually, if enough spokes disappear, the wheel might start to wobble and come clattering to a halt. About time too.

I walk on until I reach a small park. A couple are lying on the grass; she is reading, he is looking up at the inconstant clouds, coming and going in quick succession. All around me I see brightly coloured flowers. I have no idea what they are called, but it occurs to me to buy a bunch one day, perhaps only one or two, if I think the apartment needs it.

A little further on, I come to a narrow stream, too dark to gauge the depth of the water. A few steps across that little plank bridge will take me to the other side. But today is different. I back up and take a flying leap.

# THANKS

First of all, I want to thank all my fellow fearties, those people were kind enough to share their time and their insights with me, by telling their own story or describing their personal experiences of fear. A special thank you goes to Pepijn for his extraordinary open-heartedness.

Thank you to my grandmother Sjuwke, my mother Christien, and my Aunt Clara for clarifying so many things and giving me a deeper understanding of our family history.

I would also like to acknowledge the many medical professionals, academics and psychiatrists for their generosity in talking to me: Damiaan Denys, Gerrit Glas, Frans Holdert, René Kahn, Herro Kraan, Carel Manschot, Nelleke Nicolai, Miranda Olff, Jan Swinkels and Rob de Vries.

Next up are Sander Blom, Simon Dikker Hupkes, Ronald Kerstma and Nicole Lucassen of publishers Atlas Contact: thank you for welcoming me to a new home.

Thanks to my keen-eyed, ever encouraging agent Lisette Verhagen, without whom this book might never have seen the light of day.

And finally, I would like to thank Madeleijn, who has stood by me with advice, patience and love. (And continues to do so.)

If you are in need of professional help, for yourself or a loved one, make sure you get in touch with your GP.

# SOURCES

This section lists the various scientific articles and literary sources referred to in the preceding chapters, other than those for which full details have already been given.

## 2 LA VALLÉE DE MISÈRE

### On the kayaking fears of the Inuit

J.P. van Oudenhoven, *Crossculturele psychologie* [Cross-Cultural Psychology], 2002, p. 124.

### Worldwide, an estimated 7.3 per cent of people suffer from an anxiety disorder.

A.J. Baxter, K.M. Scott, T. Vos and H.A. Whiteford, "Global prevalence of anxiety disorders: a systemic review and meta-regression", *Psychological Medicine* 43, 2013, pp. 897–910.

### When we zoom out, the picture does not get any rosier.

H.U. Wittchen and F. Jacobi, "Size and burden of mental disorders in Europe – a critical review and appraisal of 27 studies", *European Neuropsychopharmacology* 15(4), 2005, pp. 357–376.

An estimated 18 per cent of the US population – some 40 million people in 2017 – are thought to be affected by an anxiety disorder in any given year.

"Past Year Prevalence of Any Anxiety Disorder Among U.S. Adults (2001–2003)", National Institute of Mental Health, nimh.nih.gov, November 2017.

J. LeDoux, *Anxious: Using the Brain to Understand and Treat Fear and Anxiety*, 2015, p. 14.

There is a neurological explanation for this [. . .] and an assumption that the consequences of those events will be disproportionately severe.

J. LeDoux, *Anxious*, 2015, pp. 97–109.

Anxious people are able to perceive threats significantly faster than people with lower levels of anxiety.

M. El Zein et al., "Anxiety dissociates the adaptive functions of sensory and motor response enhancements to social threats", *eLife* 4, 2015, pp. 1–22.

S. Kalb, *De schoonheid van angst* [The Beauty of Fear], 2019.

## 3 CHARLES DARWIN AND THE FEAR WITHIN US

Those dangers largely lose their charge as we grow older and learn to fine-tune our fears. But sometimes the tuning goes awry.

J. LeDoux, *The Emotional Brain: The Mysterious Underpinnings of Emotional Life*, 1999.

This is known as the Yerkes-Dodson law.

S. Stossel, *My Age of Anxiety. Fear, Hope, Dread and the Search for Peace of Mind*, 2014, p. 125.

R.M. Yerkes and J.D. Dodson, "The relation of strength of stimulus to rapidity of habit-formation", *Journal of Comparative Neurology and Psychology* 18(5), 1908, pp. 459–482.

**The description of how the anxious brain works is based on**

J. LeDoux, *The Emotional Brain*, 1999.

J. LeDoux, *Anxious*, 2015.

**For threat detection, the amygdala [. . .] is crucial [. . .] does not experience fear.**

S. Stossel, *My Age of Anxiety*, 2014, p. 43.

**Amygdala deficiencies have also been found in psychopaths, resulting in a dramatically tempered sense of fear and an inability to recognise or understand it in others.**

A. Marsh, *The Fear Factor: How One Emotion Connects Altruists, Psychopaths, and Everyone In-Between*, 2017.

S. Kalb, *De schoonheid van angst* [The Beauty of Fear], 2019, p. 159.

**What animals cannot do is shape or convey abstractions; even the simplest form of communication about past or future events is beyond them.**

Dutch primatologist Frans de Waal, quoted in W. Hoogendijk and W. de Rek, *Van big bang tot burn-out. Het grote verhaal over stress* [From Big Bang to Burnout: The Big Story about Stress], 2017, p. 76.

**While the primary function of the amygdala [. . .] Without a prefrontal cortex, there would be no consciousness.**

J. LeDoux, *Anxious*, 2015, p. 34.

**Many studies have shown that the amygdala [. . .] experiences no anxiety.**

J. LeDoux, *Anxious*, 2015, p. 35.

**In other words, in the dark, without any visual input, the unfortunate man felt no fear.**

The examples from Avicenna, Aquinas and Burton are given

in M.A. Lund's "Without a Cause: Fear in *The Anatomy of Melancholy*" in D. McCann, C. McKechnie-Mason (eds), *Fear in the Medical and Literary Imagination, Medieval to Modern*, 2018, pp. 37–39.

**What kind of an emotion of fear would be left [. . .] calm breathing, and a placid face?**

William James, *Psychology*, Chapter XXIV Emotion, pp. 379–380, 1892.

**It's not your tears that make you cry. . .**

This thought is taken from an essay by Dutch writer Simon Vestdijk, *Het wezen van angst* [The Essence of Fear], 1968.

**"[. . .] that which threatens cannot bring [. . .] and yet it is nowhere".**

M. Heidegger, *Being and Time*, 1962, p. 231. Translated by John Macquarrie & Edward Robinson.

**"An empty feeling in the stomach [. . .] exactly where it starts."**

G. Glas, *Concepten van angst en angststoornissen. Een psychiatrische en vakfilosofische study*. [Concepts of Anxiety and Anxiety Disorders: A Psychiatric and Professional Philosophical Study], 1991, pp. 3–6.

**A comprehensive study of Darwin's diaries, letters and documented medical history [. . .]**

S. Stossel, *My Age of Anxiety*, 2014, pp. 90–95.

## 4 THE SPELL OF THE GAMELAN

**On the English malady**

R. Hunter and I. MacAlpine, *Three Hundred Years of Psychiatry 1535–1860*, 1963.

The first usage of "neurasthenia" as a psychopathological term was by US psychiatrist E.H. Van Deusen [. . .] "excessive mental labour, especially when conjoined with anxiety".

E.H. Van Deusen, "Observations on a form of nervous prostration, (neurasthenia) culminating in insanity", *American Journal of Psychiatry* 25(4), 1869, pp. 445–461.

In the period before neurasthenia became commonly diagnosed [. . .] he had "adduced hardly any examples and quoted no statistics".

G. Berrios, *The History of Mental Symptoms. Descriptive Pyschopathology since the Nineteenth Century*, 1996, pp. 263–287.

## On Hippocrates

D. Cantor (ed.), *Reinventing Hippocrates*, 2002.

Hippocrates, *Epidemics 2 and 4–7*, Vol. VII, Loeb Classical Library 477. Translated by W. Smith, 1994.

Hippocrates, *Nature of Man. Regimen in Health. Humours. Aphorisms*, Vol. IV, Loeb Classical Library 150. Translated by W.H.S. Jones.

B. Holmes, "Disturbing Connections: Sympathetic Affections, Mental Disorder, and the Elusive Soul in Galen", in *Mental Disorders in the Classical World*, 2013, pp. 147–176.

J. Jouanna, *Hippocrates*, 1999.

E.B. Levine, *Hippocrates*, 1971.

By the eighteenth century, fear was accounting for an ever larger part of the catch-all condition of "melancholy", to the extent that leading French physician J.F. Dufour viewed "fear and sadness" as its main symptoms.

Quoted in M. Foucault, *History of Madness*, 2006, p. 263. Translated by Jonathan Murphy and Jean Khalfa.

## The quote from William Cullen

In M. Foucault, *History of Madness*, 2006, p. 324. Translated by Jonathan Murphy and Jean Khalfa.

Melancholy [. . .] was widely accepted among learned, creative and intellectual men as an unfortunate side effect of their tendency towards contemplation, and had been since the time of Aristotle.

J. Radden, *Moody Minds Distempered: Essays on Melancholy and Depression*, 2009.

**The quotes by Jaap Kunst are taken from**

His letters, the Jaap Kunst Archive, from Kunst's *Proeve van een autobiografie* [Proofs for an Autobiography] and from his granddaughter Clara Brinkgreve's *Met Indië verbonden, een verhaal van vier generaties 1849–1949* [Connected to the Indies: A Tale of Four Generations 1849–1949], 2009.

Much of the biographical information about Jaap also comes from Clara Brinkgreve's book. Personal notes and travelogues are from the Jaap Kunst Collection, part of the University of Amsterdam's Special Collections.

**Later he described their encounter: "I had travelled for days in a blacked-out train. . ."**

G. Brinkgreve, *Mozaïek van mijn leven. Herinneringen 1917–2005* [Mosaic of My Life. Memories 1917–2005], 2006, p. 61.

**"Gone were the fear and chaos. [. . .] My mother has always had two faces."**

Most of my mother's quotes are taken from S. Brinkgreve-Kunst *Ik heb ook een verhaal* [I Too Have a Story], 2008, Sjuwke's self-published memoir as told to her daughter Christien, and C. Brinkgreve *Het raadsel van goed en kwaad* [The Riddle of Good and Evil], 2018.

**On hysteria**

G. Cosmacini, *L'arte lunga. Storia della medicina dall'antichità ad oggi*, 1997.

G. Mattioli and F. Scalzone, *Attualità dell'isteria. Malattia desueta o posizione originaria?*, 2002.

H. Pérez-Rincón, "Pierre Janet, Sigmund Freud and Charcot's Psychological and Psychiatric Legacy", *Frontiers of Neurology and Neuroscience* 29, 2011, pp. 115–124.

H.E. Sigerist, *A History of Medicine. Primitive and Archaic Medicine*, 1951.

L. Sterpellone, *La Medicina Greca*, 2002.

T. Loughran, "Hysteria and neurasthenia in pre-1914 British medical discourse and in histories of shell-shock", *History of Psychiatry* 19(1), 2008, pp. 25–46.

C. Tasca et al., "Women and Hysteria in the History of Mental Health", *Clinical Practice and Epidemiology in Mental Health* 8, 2012, pp. 110–119.

**Melancholy [. . .] therefore broke up into a number of syndromes, the main one being depression.**

G.E. Berrios, "Melancholia and Depression during the 19th Century: A Conceptual History", *The British Journal of Psychiatry* 153, 1988, pp. 298–304.

**The first edition of the authoritative *Régis Practical Manual of Mental Medicine*, published in 1885, defined depression [. . .] "immobility or stupor".**

E. Régis, *A Practical Manual of Mental Medicine* (Second Edition), 1894, p. 62. Translated by H.M. Bannister.

**Physician Sir William Gull, who coined the term anorexia nervosa, wrote of mental depression "occurring without apparently adequate cause".**

W.W. Gull, *A Collection of the Published Writings of W.W. Gull*, 1894, p. 287.

Freud went on to explore the relationship between grief and melancholy but increasingly it came to be used as a vaguely descriptive term, while depression entered the medical lexicon.

R.L. Carhart-Harris et al., "Mourning and melancholia revisited: correspondences between principles of Freudian metapsychology and empirical findings in neuropsychiatry", *Annals of General Psychiatry* 7, 2008.

P. Chaslin, *Éléments de sémiologie et clinique mentales*, 1912.

A.J. Lewis, "Melancholia: A Historical Review", *Journal of Mental Science* 80, 1934, pp. 1–42.

Psychoanalysis was the method pieced together by Sigmund Freud, an approach he believed should occupy a "middle position between medicine and philosophy".

Quoted in S. Connor, *The Madness of Knowledge. On Wisdom, Ignorance and Fantasies of Knowing*, 2019, p. 99.

He saw gasping for air, a common side-effect of anxiety and panic, as a distant echo of our crying out at birth.

G. Glas, *Angst: Beleving, structuur, macht* [Fear: Perception, Structure, Power], 2001, pp. 22–30.

A contemporary and close associate of Freud, Otto Rank, went even further [. . .] by no means a recommendation.

O. Rank, *Das Trauma der Geburt und seine Bedeutung für die Psychoanalyse* [Birth Trauma and Its Implications for Psychoanalysis], 1924.

O. Rank, *Will Therapy*, 1929, p. 124. Translated by J. Taft.

## 5 BLOODLINES AND SOUNDBITES

One of the first major adoption studies was initiated in the United States in the late 1970s [. . .] nothing short of revolutionary.

S.A. Petrill et al., *Nature, Nurture, and the Transition to Early Adolescence*, 2003.

Even the time a child spent watching TV was much more consistent with the viewing habits of its biological parents than with those of its adoptive parents, though the children in the study had been less than a week old when they were given up for adoption.

R. Plomin et al., "Individual Differences in Television Viewing in Early Childhood: Nature as well as Nurture", *Psychological Science* 1, 1990, pp. 371–377.

When reunited for the first time in 1979, both brothers turned out to be six feet tall [. . .] and were father to a son.

https://science.howstuffworks.com/life/genetic/twin1.htm

These similarities went much deeper than outward appearance: reading ability, verbal skills, general learning and spatial understanding were all found to be largely genetically determined.

C.M.A. Haworth et al., "Twins Early Development Study (TEDS): A Genetically Sensitive Investigation of Cognitive and Behavioral Development from Childhood to Young Adulthood", *Twin Research and Human Genetics* 16, 2013, pp. 117–125.

According to his findings [. . .] the risk of both twins developing an anxiety disorder was [. . .] 45 compared to 15 per cent.

S. Torgersen, "Genetic factors in anxiety disorders", *Archives of General Psychiatry* 40, 1983, pp. 1085–1089.

The estimated heritability of both is between 30 and 50 per cent.

B.J. Sadock et al., *Kaplan and Sadock's Comprehensive Textbook of Psychiatry*, 2017.

The genes that affect one disorder also affect the other.

K.S. Kendler et al., "Major depression and generalized anxiety disorder. Same genes, (partly) different environments?", *Archives of General Psychiatry* 49, 1992, pp. 716–722.

N. Sartorius et al., "Depression comorbid with anxiety: results from the WHO study on psychological disorders in primary health care", *The British Journal of Psychiatry. Supplement*, 1996.

**In 1987, an influential study of 3,800 sets of Australian twins [. . .] depends on chance environmental factors.**

G. Glas, *Concepten van angst en angststoornissen. Een psychiatrische en vakfilosofische studie* [Concepts of Anxiety and Anxiety Disorders. A Psychiatric and Professional Philosophical Study], 1991, p. 107.

K.S. Kendler et al., "Symptoms of anxiety and symptoms of depression. Same genes, different environments?", *Archives of General Psychiatry* 44, 1987, pp. 451–457.

**(Previously, scientists had thought the opposite: that your chance of developing a mental illness was determined by your environment, while the form it took was genetically determined.)**

G. Carey, "Big Genes, Little Genes, Affective Disorder, and Anxiety", *Archives of General Psychiatry* 44, 1987, pp. 486–491.

**In general, you can say that experiences of loss and grief are more likely to push you towards depression, while encountering severe danger is more likely to push you towards an anxiety disorder.**

R. Finlay-Jones and G.W. Brown, "Types of stressful life event and the onset of anxiety and depressive disorders", *Psychology Medicine* 4, 1981, pp. 803–815.

**It is important to realise that no one specific gene is responsible [. . .] the OGOD misconception (one gene, one disorder).**

R. Plomin et al., "The Genetic Basis of Complex Human Behaviors", *Science* 264, 1994, pp. 1733–1739.

**The brother dilemma outlined comes from**

R. Plomin, *Blueprint: How DNA Makes Us Who We Are*, 2018, pp. 75–85.

**And is further supported by**

J. Dunn and R. Plomin, *Separate Lives: Why Siblings Are So Different*, 1990.

D. Reiss et al., *The Relationship Code: Deciphering Genetic and Social Influences on Adolescent Development*, 2000.

A. Pike et al., "Family environment and adolescent depressive symptoms and antisocial behavior. A multivariate genetic analysis", *Developmental Psychology* 32, 1996, pp. 590–603.

**A mother is often overprotective of an anxious child, and this can lead the father to compensate subconsciously by being stricter.**

I.E. Lindhout et al., "Childrearing Style in Families of Anxiety-Disordered Children: Between-Family and Within-Family Differences", *Child Psychiatry and Human Development* 40, 2009, pp. 197–212.

**Rats that were frequently licked and stroked by their mothers [. . .] genes in the hippocampus.**

I.C.G. Weaver, "Life at the Interface Between a Dynamic Environment and a Fixed Genome: Epigenetic Programming of Stress Responses by Maternal Behavior", in D. Janigro (ed.), *Mammalian Brain Development*, 2009, pp. 17–39. Quoted in: J. De Mul, "Survival of the fittest metaphor", afterword to the Dutch translation of D. Noble, *The Music of Life*, 2016, p. 198.

**Mice whose cages contained toys when they were young gave birth to offspring with more highly developed cognitive functions.**

J.A. Arai et al., "Transgenerational Rescue of a Genetic Defect in Long-Term Potentiation and Memory Formation by Juvenile Enrichment", *Journal of Neuroscience* 5, 2009, pp. 1496–1502.

**An extensive Swedish study [. . .]**

M.E. Pembrey et al., "Sex-specific, Male-Line Transgenerational Responses in Humans", *European Journal of Human Genetics* 14, 2006, pp. 159–166. Quoted in: J. De Mul, "Survival of the fittest metaphor", afterword to the Dutch translation of D. Noble, *The Music of Life*, 2016, p. 198.

**A study of the male children of soldiers [. . .] in the American Civil War found that they were 10 per cent more likely to die in any given year on reaching middle age.**

B. Carey, "Can We Really Inherit Trauma?", *The New York Times*, 10 December 2018.

**Another American study concluded that Dutch people whose foetal development [. . .] made them relatively overweight later in life.**

B.T. Heijmans et al., "Persistent Epigenetic Differences Associated with Prenatal Exposure to Famine in Humans", *Proceedings of the National Academy of Sciences of the United States of America* 105(44), 2008, pp. 17046–17049.

**It has taught me that the division of human experience into environmental factors and the genetic component is largely artificial.**

A. Marsman et al., "Do Current Measures of Polygenic Risk for Mental Disorders Contribute to Population Variance in Mental Health?", *Schizophrenia Bulletin*, 16 July 2020.

## 6 THE BAT'S DARK SHADOW

**My experience of the world was characterised by an inability to impose order.**

The correspondence between this perception and an anxiety profile is pointed out in G. Glas, *Concepten van angst en angststoornissen* [Concepts of Anxiety and Anxiety Disorders], 1991, p. 33.

**"Daan is a very intense child,"** my mother, then a sociology professor, said in a 1997 interview.

These quotes come from an interview in *Marie Claire* by Elisabeth Lockhorn, in March 1997, and have been lightly edited with my mother's approval.

## The passages on attachment

*This American Life*, "Unconditional Love", Episode 317.

J. Bowlby, *Maternal Care and Mental Health*, 1950.

J. Bowlby and M. Fry (eds), *Child Care and the Growth of Love*, 1965.

J. Bowlby, *Attachment and Loss: Vol. 1. Attachment*, 1969.

J. Bowlby, *Separation: Anxiety & Anger*, 1973.

G. van Egmond, *Bodemloos bestaan. Problemen met adoptiekinderen* [Bottomless Existence. Problems with Adopted Children], 2007.

E. Galinsky, "Trusting Relationships Are Central to Children's Learning – Lessons from Edward Tronick", *Huffington Post*, 6 December 2017.

M. Robinson, *Understanding Behaviour and Development in Early Childhood: A Guide to Theory and Practice*, 2011, p. 48.

N.P. Rygaard, *Hechtingsstoornissen* [Attachment Disorders], 2007.

S. Stossel, *My Age of Anxiety*, 2014, pp. 245–255.

E. Tronick, *The Neurobehavioral and Social-Emotional Development of Infants and Children*, 2007.

## The passages on Panksepp

J. Panksepp, *Affective Neuroscience: The Foundations of Human and Animal Emotions*, 1998.

J. Panksepp (ed.), *A Textbook of Biological Psychiatry*, 2004.

J. Panksepp and L. Biven, *The Archaeology of Mind: Neuroevolutionary Origins of Human Emotions*, 2012.

A conversation with psychiatrist Ariette van Reekum and child psychiatrist Marcel Smeets, 22 February 2019.

Roughly speaking, if you feel unsafe in your attachment and never really learn to put your trust in others, you will be more inclined towards panic.

F. Boer, *Angst. Van monster tot stille kracht* [Fear: From Monster to Silent Force], 2018, p. 102.

Looking back on his years as a bat, Adam West mused that everyone wanted to be Batman [. . .] we all have something of the avenger, the vigilante in us.

Extras from *Batman: The Complete Television Series* (DVD), 2015.

For the life story of Bruce Wayne/Batman, I drew on several sources.

G. Johns, *Flashpoint*, 2011.

S. Liu and L. Montgomery, *Batman: Year One*, 2011, animated film.

F. Miller, *Batman: Year One*, 1987.

C. Nolan, *Batman Begins*, 2005, film.

C. Nolan, *The Dark Knight*, 2008, film.

C. Nolan, *The Dark Knight Rises*, 2012, film.

J. Schumacher, *Batman Forever* (out-takes), 1995, film.

J. Todd, "Dreaming the Bat out of the Shadow", *Psychological Perspectives* 59, 2016, pp. 219–241.

M.D. White and R. Arp (eds), *Batman and Philosophy: The Dark Knight of the Soul*, 2008.

"Batman: Facing Your Fear and Anger Constructively", *Pop Mythology*, 1 March 2011.

The passages on Kierkegaard

W. Ietswaart, "Vrijheid en angst. Over Kierkegaards angsttheorie" [Freedom and Fear. On Kierkegaard's Theory of Fear], *Tijdschrijft voor Pyschoanalyse* 8, 2002, p. 2.

S. Kierkegaard, *Fear and Trembling*, 1843. Translated by W. Lowrie, 1941.

S. Kierkegaard, *The Concept of Anxiety*, 1844. Edited and translated by Reidar Thomte in collaboration with Albert B. Anderson, 1980.

S. Kierkegaard, *The Sickness unto Death*, 1849. Edited and translated by Howard V. Hong and Edna H. Hong, 1980.

J. Mommers, "De Socrates van Kopenhagen" [The Socrates of Copenhagen], *De Groene Amsterdammer*, 1 May 2013.

A. Visser, *Kierkegaard en het begrip angst, een leesgids* [Kierkegaard and the Concept of Fear: A Reader's Guide], 2018.

**This idea is akin to what psychoanalyst Otto Rank called "fear of life" [. . .] finding a balance and accepting them both.**

R. May, *The Meaning of Anxiety*, 1950.

S. Kalb, *De schoonheid van angst* [The Beauty of Fear], 2019, pp. 94–95.

**The passages on Heidegger**

M. Heidegger, *Being and Time*, 1927. Translated by John Macquarrie & Edward Robinson, 1962.

S. Vestdijk, *Het wezen van de angst* [The Essence of Fear], 1968, pp. 381–390.

M.D. White and R. Arp (eds), *Batman and Philosophy: The Dark Knight of the Soul*, 2008.

J. van Sluis, *Leeswijzer bij Zijn en Tijd* [Being and Time: A Reader's Guide], 1998.

**The quote from Jung**

C. Jung, *Psychology and Religion*, 1938, *Collected Works* 11, p. 131.

**Biologists distinguish between two types of aggression [. . .] drowns out the stress hormone we call cortisol.**

W. Hoogendijk and W. de Rek, *Van big bang tot burn-out. Het grote verhaal over stress* [From Big Bang to Burnout: The Big Story about Stress], 2017, pp. 173–176.

**Gaupp's research on Ernst August Wagner**

R. Gaupp, *Zur Psychologie des Massenmords: Hauptlehrer Wagner von Degerloch* [On the Psychology of Mass Murder: Headteacher Wagner from Degerloch], 1914.

R. Gaupp, "Der Fall Wagner. Eine Katamnese, zugleich ein Beitrag zur Lehre von der Paranoia" [The Case of Wagner: A Catamnesis and a Contribution to the Theory of Paranoia], *Zeitschrift für die gesamte Neurologie und Psychiatrie*, 60, 1920, pp. 312–327.

R. van Raden, *Patient Massenmörder. Der Fall Ernst Wagner und die biopolitischen Diskurse* [Patient, Mass Murderer: The Case of Ernst Wagner and the Biopolitical Discourses], 2009.

**The passage on Anders Breivik**

B. Amland and S. Dilorenzo, "Norway suspect wanted European anti-Muslim crusade", *The Washington Times*, 24 July 2011.

M. Goldberg, "Norway Massacre: Anders Breivik's Deadly Attack Fueled by Hatred of Women", *The Daily Beast*, 24 July 2011.

J.C. Jones, "Anders Breivik's chilling antifeminism", *The Guardian*, 27 July 2011.

J. Pappas, "Cultural Genocide", libertyandculture.blogspot.com, 25 July 2011.

Å. Seierstad, *One of Us: The Story of Anders Breivik and the Massacre in Norway*. Translated by Sarah Death, 2015.

**The manifesto attributed to Crusius**

Y. Aboutaleb, "What's inside the hate-filled manifesto linked to the alleged El Paso shooter", *The Washington Post*, 4 August 2019

https://randallpacker.com/wp-content/uploads/2019/08/The-Inconvenient-Truth.pdf

**Aristotle's three conditions**
Quoted in M.C. Nussbaum, *The Monarchy of Fear: A Philosopher Looks at Our Political Crisis*, 2018.

**The collection that features the Anna Enquist poem**
C. Dresselhuys & J. Wesselius (eds), *Vrouwentroost* [Female Consolation], 1994.

## 7 BIRTH OF AN ILLNESS

**On Alice Neville**
A. Neville, *Who's Afraid of Agoraphobia? Facing Up to Fear and Anxiety*, 1986.
A. Neville, *No Fear. Overcoming Panic Attacks and Phobias*, 2003.

**On The Open Door**
I.M. Marks and E.R. Herst, "A Survey of 1,200 Agoraphobics in Britain: Features Associated with Treatment and Ability to Work", *Social Psychiatry* 5(1), 1970, pp. 16–24.

**As strange as some of these phobias sound [. . .] can lead to rejection by the group.**
W. Gomperts, *De opkomst van de sociale fobie. Een sociologische en psychologische studie naar de maatschappelijke verandering van psychische verschijnselen* [The Rise of Social Phobia. A Sociological and Psychological Study of the Social Change of Mental Phenomena], 1992, pp. 61–64.

**To this day, women are one and a half times more likely to be diagnosed with an anxiety disorder than men, regardless of age group.**
R. de Graaf et al., "Incidentie van psychische aandoeningen. Opzet en eerste resultaten van de tweede meting van de studie NEMESIS-2" [Incidence of Mental Disorders. Design and Initial

Results of the Second Measurement of the NEMESIS-2 Study], Trimbos Institute, 2012.

G. Glas, *Concepten van angst en angststoornissen. Een psychiatrische en vakfilosofische study.* [Concepts of Anxiety and Anxiety Disorders: A Psychiatric and Professional Philosophical Study], 1991.

**A 2014 study conducted by Florida State University biomedical scientist Mohamed Kabbaj concluded that testosterone [. . .] as a neurological buffer against anxiety.**

J. McHenry et al., "Sex Differences in Anxiety and Depression: Role of Testosterone", *Frontiers in Neuroendocrinology* 35(1), 2014, pp. 42–57.

**Meanwhile, the hormones oestrogen and progesterone [. . .] even when a threat has been shown not to be genuine.**

Science magazine *Wetenschap in beeld* 12, 2020, p. 19.

**The only researcher to make a serious attempt to explain the difference between men and women with respect to [agoraphobia] was sociologist Abram de Swaan.**

A. de Swaan, *De draagbare De Swaan* [The Portable De Swaan], 1999, pp. 151–163.

**On the life and work of Cicero**

M. Bento, "The Exile of Marcus Tullius Cicero: From Savior to Shame", written for the course *Introduction to Historical Research* at CUNY, 18 December 2014.

Cicero, *Back from Exile: Six Speeches upon His Return.* Translated with introduction and notes by D.R. Shackleton Bailey, 1991.

Cicero, *Cicero on the Emotions: Tusculan Disputations 3 and 4.* Translated with commentary by M. Graver, 2001.

Cicero, *The Letters of Cicero: The Whole Extant Correspondence in Chronological Order.* Vol. 1, 1899. Translated by E.S. Shuckburgh.

Cicero, *Tusculan Disputations*, Loeb Classical Library 141. Translated by J.E. King, 1927.

A. Everitt, *Cicero: The Life and Times of Rome's Greatest Politician*, 2001.

H.J. Haskell, *This Was Cicero*, 1964.

D. den Hengst and W. Kassies, *Brieven van Cicero* [Letters of Cicero], 1985.

E. Narducci, "Perceptions of Exile in Cicero: The Philosophical Interpretation of a Real Experience", *American Journal of Philology* 118(1), 1997, pp. 55–73.

H.C. Nutting, "Cicero in Exile", *The Classical Weekly* 23(22), 1930, p. 176.

Plutarch, *Life of Caesar*. Translated by R. Warner.

M.V. Root, "A Visit to Cicero's Tusculanum", *The Classical Journal* 16(1), 1920, pp. 34–41.

## On Epicurus

Lucretius, *The Way Things Are: The De Rerum Natura*, Book VI, pp. 14–16, 24–27. Translated by R. Humphries, 1968.

## On Seneca

Seneca, *De tranquillitate animi*, ch. 11. Translated by J.W. Basore, 1932.

Seneca, *De brevitate vitae*, ch. 15. Translated by G.D. Williams, 2003.

Seneca, *Brieven aan Lucilius* [Letters to Lucilius]. Translated by C. Verhoeven, 1980, p. 22.

Seneca, *Letters from a Stoic*. Translated by R. Campbell, 2004. The quote from Seneca is from the translation by Richard M. Gummere, 1917.

## On Epictetus and Spinoza

S. Stossel, *My Age of Anxiety*, 2014, pp. 12–13 and pp. 110–111.

The quote from Epictetus is based on the translation by Thomas Wentworth Higginson, 1964.

### The passages on Little Albert

N. Digdona et al., "Watson's Alleged Little Albert Scandal: Historical Breakthrough or New Watson Myth?", *Revista de Historia de la Psicología* 35(1), 2014, pp. 47–60.

J.B. Watson and J.J.B. Morgan, "Emotional Reactions and Psychological Experimentation", *The American Journal of Psychology* 28(2), 1917, pp. 163–174.

J.B. Watson and R. Rayner, "Conditioned Emotional Reactions", *Journal of Experimental Psychology*, 3(1), 1920, pp. 1–14.

M.N. de Wolf-Ferdinandusse and E.J. Zwaan, *Leven met angst* [Living with Fear], 1981, p. 24.

### The passages on cognitive behavioural therapy

K. Oatley, *Emotions: A Brief History*, 2004, p. 53.

G.L. Thorpe and S.L. Olson, *Behavior Therapy: Concepts, Procedures, and Applications*, 1997.

## 8 PANDORA'S BOXES

### The passages on Kraepelin

M. Brüne, "On Human Self-domestication, Psychiatry, and Eugenics", *Philosophy, Ethics, and Humanities in Medicine* 2:21, 2007.

E.J. Engstrom, "'On the Question of Degeneration' by Emil Kraepelin (1908)1", *History of Psychiatry*, 18(3), 2007, pp. 389–398.

E.J. Engstrom et al., "Emil Wilhelm Magnus Georg Kraepelin (1856–1926)", *American Journal of Psychiatry* 163(10), 2006, p. 1710.

H. Hippius et al., *The University Department of Psychiatry in*

Munich. *From Kraepelin and his Predecessors to Molecular Psychiatry*, 2007.

L.R. Mandlis, *The (Un)Usual Body: Foundational Transphobia in Psychiatry, Law, and Citizenship*, 2011.

## The passages on the origins of the DSM

M.A. Crocq, "A History of Anxiety: From Hippocrates to DSM", *Dialogues in Clinical Neuroscience* 17(3), 2015, pp. 319–325.

G.N. Grob, "The Origins of American Psychiatric Epidemiology", *American Journal of Public Health* 75(3), 1985, pp. 229–236.

G.N. Grob, "Origins of DSM-I: A Study in Appearance and Reality", *American Journal of Psychiatry*, 148(4), 1991, pp. 421–431.

A.V. Horwith, *Anxiety. A Short History*, 2013.

A.C. Houts, "Fifty years of psychiatric nomenclature: reflections on the 1943 War Department Technical Bulletin, Medical 203", *Journal of Clinical Psychology*, 56(7), 2000, pp. 935–967.

W.C. Menninger, "The relationship of clinical psychology and psychiatry", *American Psychologist* 5(1), 1950, pp. 3–15.

## The passages on DSM III

Darian Leader's quote about Cinderella's slipper comes from *What Is Madness*, 2011, p. 27.

P.J. Caplan, *They Say You're Crazy. How the World's Most Powerful Psychiatrists Decide Who's Normal*, 1995.

J. Davies, "How Voting and Consensus Created the Diagnostic and Statistical Manual of Mental Disorders (DSM-III)", *Anthropology & Medicine* 24(1), 2017, pp. 32–46.

H.S. Decker, *The Making of DSM-III®: A Diagnostic Manual's Conquest of American Psychiatry*, 2013.

G. Glas, *Concepten van angst en angststoornissen. Een psychiatrische en vakfilosofische study.* [Concepts of Anxiety and Anxiety Disorders: A Psychiatric and Professional Philosophical Study], 1991, pp. 100–105.

G. Glas, *Angst: Beleving, structuur, macht* [Fear: Perception, Structure, Power], 2008, pp. 28–29.

C. Lane, *Shyness: How Normal Behaviour Became a Sickness*, 2007.

C. Lane, "Are We Really That Ill?", *The New York Sun*, 26 March 2008.

C. Lane, "Wrangling over psychiatry's bible", *Los Angeles Times*, 16 November 2008.

S. Stossel, *My Age of Anxiety*, 2014, pp. 180–200.

**David Sheehan on the DSM dinner discussions**

S. Stossel, *My Age of Anxiety*, 2014, p. 193.

**Compare DSM IV to the document at the root of it all – the original Medical 203 – and the number of psychiatric diagnoses is a staggering 800 per cent higher.**

A.C. Houts, "Fifty years of psychiatric nomenclature: reflections on the 1943 War Department Technical Bulletin, Medical 203", *Journal of Clinical Psychology*, 56(7), 2000, pp. 935–967.

**This point was neatly made by psychologist Paul Verhaeghe when he proposed that Mania Diagnostica Activa (MDA) – or diagnosis mania – be granted official DSM recognition.**

S. Bloemink, *Diagnosedrift. Hoe onze labelcultuur kinderen tekort doet* [Diagnosis Mania. How Our Label Culture Shortchanges Children], 2018, p. 8.

**Under the DSM regime, the main currency consists of semicoincidental labels [. . .] have done little to change this situation.**

M. Vermeulen, *"Last van het verkeerde label"* [Burden of the Wrong Label], *de Volkskrant*, 23 January 2021.

**But often corporate influence is more nebulous, as in the case of industry-sponsored "ambassadors" or "key opinion leaders".**

R. Feldman, *Drugs, Money, and Secret Handshakes. The Unstoppable Growth of Prescription Drug Prices*, 2018.

**Similar climate fears exist today, of course, often in intensified form.**

J. Smit, "Klimaatangst: stress, shocks en identiteitsverlies door klimaatverandering" [Climate Anxiety: Stress, Shocks and Identity Loss from Climate Change], *HP/De Tijd*, 29 August 2019.

A. Mooij, *Geslachtsziekten en besmettingsangst. Een historischsociologische studie, 1850–1990* [Sexually Transmitted Diseases and Fear of Contagion. A Historical-Sociological Study, 1850–1990], 1993.

W.H. McNeill, *Plagues and Peoples*, 1976.

**About the looping effect**

T. Dehue, *De depressie-epidemie* [The Depression Epidemic], 2010.

I. Hacking, "Making Up People" in T.C. Heller, M. Sosna and D.E. Wellbery (ed.), *Reconstructing Individualism*, 1986, pp. 161–171.

I. Hacking, "The Making and Molding of Child Abuse", *Critical Inquiry* 17(2), 1991, pp. 253–288.

I. Hacking, "The Looping Effects of Human Kinds", in D. Sperber, D. Premack and A.J. Premack (eds), *Causal Cognition: A Multidisciplinary Debate*, 1995, pp. 351–383.

I. Hacking, "Making Up People", *London Review of Books*, 17 August 2006.

The quote from Damiaan Denys is from a conversation I had with him in July 2019.

The quote from Jan Swinkels is from a conversation I had with him in November 2018.

**For every hundred Dutch people who had an anxiety disorder in 1992, there were four hundred and fifty in 2010, according to Maastricht University's Research Network on Family Medicine.**

T.S. Brugha et al., "Trends in Service Use and Treatment for Mental Disorders in Adults throughout Great Britain", *British Journal of Psychiatry*, 185(5), 2004, pp. 378–384.

R. de Graaf et al., "Incidentie van psychische aandoeningen. Opzet en eerste resultaten van de tweede meting van de studie NEMESIS-2" [Incidence of Mental Disorders. Design and Initial Results of the Second Measurement of the NEMESIS-2 Study], Trimbos Institute, 2012.

R. Jenkins et al., "The National Psychiatric Morbidity Surveys of Great Britain: Initial Findings from the Household Survey", *Psychological Medicine* 27(4), 1997, pp. 775–789.

R.C. Kessler and T.B. Üstün, "The World Health Organization Composite International Diagnostic Interview", in R.C. Kessler and T.B. Üstün (eds), *The WHO World Mental Health Surveys: Global Perspectives on the Epidemiology of Mental Disorders*, 2008, pp. 58–90.

Figures obtained by the Trimbos Institute, following a comparison between their large-scale study NEMESIS 1 (1996–1999) and NEMESIS 2 (2007–2018).

**Worldwide, estimates by the World Health Organization point to a 15 per cent rise the number of people with anxiety disorders over the past decade.**

Science magazine *Wetenschap in beeld* 12, 2020, p. 18.

**"The difference between domestic animals and livestock raised for slaughter may be arbitrary – for sacred cows, you need only go to India – but it pretty much determines their fate."**

Professor Trudy Dehue in conversation at Amsterdam's Arti et Amicitiae society on 13 February 2019.

SSRIs accounted for more than half of the over one million anti-depressants prescribed in the Netherlands in 2017.

Source: the Dutch Foundation for Pharmaceutical Statistics (SFK).

The first barbiturate was produced in 1864 by a German chemist [. . .] marketed to humans.

S. Stossel, *My Age of Anxiety*, 2014, p. 157.

In 1951, *The New York Times* described barbiturates as "more of a menace to society than heroin or morphine".

S. Stossel, *My Age of Anxiety*, 2014, p. 158.

In 1954, Marthe Vogt, a German neuroscientist working in the UK, discovered the role that norepinephrine (also known as noradrenaline) [. . .] plays as a neurotransmitter.

S. Stossel, *My Age of Fear*, 2014, pp. 170–180.

In 1957, pharmaceutical company Hoffmann-La Roche marketed iproniazid, under the trade name Marsilid, one of the world's first antidepressants.

S. Stossel, *My Age of Anxiety*, 2014, pp. 160–170.

About the TB ward in New Jersey

J. Hari, *Lost Connections. Why You're Depressed and How to Find Hope*, 2018, pp. 33–34.

S. Stossel, *My Age of Anxiety*, 2014, pp. 170–180.

In September 1959, *The New York Times* published an article about Marsilid and the first tricylic drugs, describing them as "anti-depressants" – a brand-new term at the time.

S. Stossel, *My Age of Anxiety*, 2014, p. 178.

The 1970s brought the fourth (and to date final) wave of pharmacological breakthroughs in the field of anti-anxiety medication: the advent of the SSRI.

J. LeDoux, *Anxious*, 2015, pp. 104–106, 238–244.

**Michel Houellebecq on serotonin and amoebae**

From Houellebecq's novel *Serotonin*, 2019, p. 80. Translation by Shaun Whiteside.

For the sake of readability in context, I have taken the liberty of rendering this excerpt in the present tense, with the added justification that the original is written in the past tense but set in the future.

SSRIs have gradually come to dominate the market in antidepressants. Antibiotics aside, they are thought to be the best-selling drugs in the history of the world.

S. Stossel, *My Age of Anxiety*, 2014, p. 211.

Ronald Pies, former editor of the magazine *Psychiatric Times*, describes the term chemical imbalance as "a kind of bumper-sticker term that saves time".

R. Aviv, "The Challenge of Going Off Psychiatric Drugs", *The New Yorker*, 1 April 2019.

[. . .] that finely tuned system of some 450,000 kilometres of wiring, with between five and ten thousand trillion interconnections [. . .]

Conversations with Jan Swinkels, October 2018.

[. . .] the focus now was on obtaining facts and generating data, taking an evidence-based, demonstrably scientific approach.

P. Verhaeghe, *Identiteit* [Identity], 2012, p. 75.

Kahn estimated that around 60 per cent of patients would show an immediate response.

P. Witteman, *Opgenomen. Witteman bij de psychiater* [Committed. Witteman at the Psychiatrist's], 1997, p. 144.

**"The point is that psychiatry, like the rest of the medical world, is now becoming scientific and measurable. In the past, it was too much of an art, a philosophy."**

Quoted in A. Schipper, "De psychiater is optimistisch" [The psychiatrist is optimistic], *Trouw*, 22 June 1995.

**Damien Denys on patients and patience**

Quote noted during an interview on 7 July 2019.

**The full extent of this practice was only studied for the first time recently, by law professor Robin Feldman.**

R. Feldman, *Drugs, Money and Secret Handshakes*, 2018.

**Former GP and renowned epidemiologist Dick Bijl begs to differ.**

All quotations by Dick Bijl are from M. Finoulst, "We slikken te veel pillen" [We take too many pills], *Knack*, 19 August 2018 and D. Bijl, *Het pillenprobleem. Waarom we zoveel medicijnen gebruiken die niet werken en niet helpen* [The Pill Problem. Why We Take So Many Drugs that Don't Work and Don't Help], 2018.

**In his view, many such studies are rush jobs [. . .] that are poorly conducted.**

D. Bijl, *Het pillenprobleem* [The Pill Problem], pp. 15–18.

R. Aviv, "The Challenge of Going Off Psychiatric Drugs", *The New Yorker*, 1 April 2019.

**Of all the drug studies conducted by pharmaceutical companies, up to 40 per cent have never been released at all, while the remaining 60 per cent are subject to highly selective publication practices.**

J. Hari, *Lost Connections*, 2018, p. 28

[. . .] psychiatrist Bram Bakker said " [. . .] were not included in the study."

From a 2009 interview for *Kijken in de ziel*, a series of in-depth TV interviews with leading Dutch psychiatrists and pyschologists.

The history of the world's most famous antidepressant, Prozac, is a case in point.

J. Hari, *Lost Connections*, 2018, pp. 28–29.

Professor Irving Kirsch of Harvard Medical School [. . .] only marginally better than those given placebos.

I. Kirsch and G. Sapirstein, "Listening to Prozac but Hearing Placebo: A Meta-analysis of Antidepressant Medication", *Prevention & Treatment* 1(2), 26 June 1998.

"One thing I do pride myself on," he later told British journalist Johann Hari, "is looking at the data, and allowing my mind to be changed when the data's different than I expected."

J. Hari, *Lost Connections*, 2018, p. 30.

Following an additional study in 2008, Kirsch found that the pills work primarily in patients with a very severe depressive disorder.

Quoted in D. Bijl, *Het pillenprobleem* [The Pill Problem], p. 107.

[. . .] leading American neuroscientist Joseph LeDoux cites another fundamental reason for their shortcomings: antidepressants essentially dampen our responses without removing our anxiety.

J. LeDoux in the *The Joe Rogan Experience* podcast, episode 1344, 5 September 2019.

J. LeDoux, *Anxious*, 2015, pp. 104–106, 238–244.

[. . .] this is a crude and inaccurate indiscriminate [. . .] memory and attention.

J. LeDoux in the *The Joe Rogan Experience* podcast, episode 1344, 5 September 2019.

**In fact, most studies show that CBT is about as effective as medication when it comes to anxiety disorders, but with less chance of relapse.**

B. Bandelow et al., "Meta-analysis of Randomized Controlled Comparisons of Psychopharmacological and Psychological Treatments for Anxiety Disorders", *World Journal of Biological Psychiatry* 8(3), 2007, pp. 175–187.

S. Blomhoff et al., "Randomised Controlled General Practice Trial of Sertraline, Exposure Therapy and Combined Treatment in Generalised Social Phobia", *British Journal of Psychiatry* 179(1), 2001, pp. 23–30.

D.M. Clark et al., "Cognitive Therapy versus Fluoxetine in Generalized Social Phobia: A Randomized Placebo-controlled Trial", *Journal of Consulting and Clinical Psychology* 71(6), 2003, pp. 1058–1067.

J.R. Davidson, "Pharmacotherapy of Social Anxiety Disorder: What Does the Evidence Tell Us?", *Journal of Clinical Psychiatry* 67 (suppl. 12), 2006, pp. 20–26.

T.A. Furukawa et al., "Combined Psychotherapy plus Antidepressants for Panic Disorder with or without Agoraphobia", *Cochrane Database of Systematic Reviews* 004364, 2007.

V. Hunot et al., "Psychological Therapies for Generalized Anxiety Disorder", *Cochrane Database of Systematic Reviews* 001848, 2007.

K. Mitte, "A Meta-analysis of the Efficacy of Psycho- and Pharmacotherapy in Panic Disorder with and without Agoraphobia", *Journal of Affective Disorders* 88(1), 2005, pp. 27–45.

P.J. Norton and E.C. Price, "A Meta-analytic Review of Adult Cognitive-Behavioral Treatment Outcome across Anxiety Disorders", *Journal of Nervous and Mental Disease* 195(6), 2007, pp. 521–531.

## On Jean Twenge's research

A.T. Beck, "Theoretical Perspectives on Clinical Anxiety", in A. Hussain Tuma and J.D. Maser (eds), *Anxiety and the Anxiety Disorders*, 1985, pp. 183–196.

S. Torgersen, "Relationship between Adult and Childhood Anxiety Disorders: Genetic Hypothesis" in C. Last (ed.), *Anxiety Across the Lifespan: A Developmental Perspective*, 1993, pp. 113–127.

J.M. Twenge, "The Age of Anxiety? Birth Cohort Change in Anxiety and Neuroticism, 1952–1993", *Journal of Personality and Social Psychology* 79(6), 2000, pp. 1007–1021.

J.M. Twenge and W.K. Campbell, *The Narcissism Epidemic: Living in the Age of Entitlement*, 2009.

J.M. Twenge, *Generation Me: Why Today's Young Americans are More Confident, Assertive, Entitled – and More Miserable Than Ever Before*, 2014.

**(Some philosophers have referred to the period of relative calm [. . .] as the *interanxietas* or interbellum of fear.)**

R. Riemen, "A New Age of Anxiety", Introductory Essay for the 2020 Nexus Conference.

## 10 FROM SOLIDARITY TO SOLITARY

### Dirk van der Zee on football clubs and individualism

M. Dekker, "Hoe moet de club draaien zonder zijn vrijwilligers?" [How is a club supposed to run without its volunteers?], *NRC Handelsblad*, 8 March 2017.

**In 1950, nine per cent of Americans lived alone; in 2010 that figure was twenty-eight per cent.**

J.M. Twenge, *Generation Me*, 2014, p. 155.

**In 1947, there were three hundred thousand one-person households in the Netherlands; today there are three million.**

H. Boersma, "*Modernisering is de weg naar een beter leven*" [Modernisation is the way to a better life], *De Groene Amsterdammer*, 15 August 2018.

**You are almost twice as likely to have an anxiety disorder if you live alone than if you cohabit.**

R. de Graaf, M. ten Have, M. Tuithof and S. van Dorsselaer, "*Incidentie van psychische aandoeningen. Opzet en eerste resultaten van de tweede meting van de studie NEMESIS-2*" [Incidence of Mental Illness. Design and Initial Results of the Second Measurement of the NEMESIS-2 Study], Trimbos Institute, 2012.

**Recent follow-up reseach has shown this to be a matter of causation rather than simple correlation. [. . .] People who do not have a mental health problem [. . .] substance abuse within a number of years.**

J. Nuyen et al., "The bidirectional relationship between loneliness and common mental disorders in adults: findings from a longitudinal population-based cohort study", *Social Psychiatry and Psychiatric Epidemiology* 55(10), 2019, pp. 1297–1310.

**You are also almost twice as likely to have an anxiety disorder if you live in a big city [. . .]**

R. de Graaf et al., "*Incidentie van psychische aandoeningen. Opzet en eerste resultaten van de tweede meting van de studie NEMESIS-2*" [Incidence of Mental Illness. Design and Initial Results of the Second Measurement of the NEMESIS-2 Study], Trimbos Institute, 2012.

**On the religious front: in 2018, Statistics Netherlands reported [. . .] for 46 per cent of the population.**

Quoted in M. Pam, "Hoe God verdween uit Nederland" [How

God Disappeared from the Netherlands], *HP/De Tijd*, December 2018.

**The conclusion of a 2008 study on social cohesion in the Netherlands, the largest in the country to date, pulled no punches [. . .]**

P. Schnabel, R. Bijl and J. de Hart, *Betrekkelijke betrokkenheid: Studies in sociale cohesie* [Relative Involvement: Studies in Social Cohesion], report by The Netherlands Institute for Social Research, 2008.

**There is a direct link between social cohesion and how happy people are with the circumstances in which they live: the greater the social cohesion in a neighbourhood, a city or a country, the happier and less anxious people are.**

*De sociale staat van Nederland* [The Social State of the Netherlands], report by The Netherlands Institute for Social Research, 2017.

**A more appealing but less common term for social cohesion is "art of association", coined by political scientist Francis Fukuyama.**

Francis Fukuyama, *Trust: The Social Virtues & The Creation of Prosperity*, 1995.

**Sociologist Émile Durkheim referred to this state of increasing disorientation as "anomie".**

Quoted in A. de Swaan, *De draagbare De Swaan* [The Portable De Swaan], 1999, p. 152.

**Gerrit Wagner's quote on winners and losers**

F. Milikowski, *Een klein land met verre uithoeken. Ongelijke kansen in veranderend Nederland* [A Small Country with Distant Corners. Unequal Opportunities in the Changing Netherlands], 2020.

**Margaret Thatcher's quotes on society and the soul**

*The Sunday Times*, 3 May 1981 and *Woman's Own*, 23 September 1987.

**In the absence of competing ideologies or systems, the market economy gradually led to a market society, to borrow a description from Harvard philosopher Michael Sandel.**

From M.J. Sandel, *The Tyranny of Merit: What's Become of the Common Good?*, 2020.

**Whereas in 1964 only 29 per cent of American voters believed that the government was "pretty much run by a few big interests. . ." by 2013 the view [. . .] was held by 79 per cent.**

D. Cole, "How Corrupt Are Our Politics?", *The New York Review of Books*, 25 September 2014.

T.B. Edsall, "The Value of Political Corruption", *The New York Times*, 5 August 2014.

**On economic conditions and fear**

W. Davies, *Nervous States. How Feeling Took Over the World*, 2018.

J.M. Twenge, "The Age of Anxiety? Birth Cohort Change in Anxiety and Neuroticism, 1952–1993", *Journal of Personality and Social Psychology* 79(6), 2000, pp. 1007–1021.

P. Verhaeghe, *Identiteit* [Identity], 2012, pp. 189–195.

R. Wilkinson and K. Pickett (eds), *Health and Inequality (Major Themes in Health and Social Welfare)*, 2008.

R. Wilkinson and K. Pickett, *The Spirit Level: Why More Equal Societies Almost Always Do Better*, 2009.

R. Wilkinson and K. Pickett, *The Inner Level: How More Equal Societies Reduce Stress, Restore Sanity and Improve Everyone's Well-Being*, 2018.

**Will Davies's findings about income**

W. Davies, *Nervous States. How Feeling Took Over the World*

(2018), quoted in N. van Verschuer, "Hoe angst de wereld ver-overde" [How fear took over the world], in *NRC Handelsblad*, 27 September 2018.

**This is emblematic of a wider picture that holds true for all neoliberal-led countries [. . .]**

B. van Bavel and E. Frankema, "Wealth Inequality in the Neth-erlands, c. 1950–2015. The Paradox of a Northern European Welfare State", *TSEG/Low Countries Journal of Social and Eco-nomic History* 14(2), 2017, pp. 29–62.

Statistics Netherlands, *Een eeuw in statistieken* [A Century in Statistics], 2010.

**[. . .] Italian philosopher Paolo Virno argues that today's Western economies are sustained by a growing precariat [. . .]**

Paolo Virno is quoted in J. Hari, *Lost Connections*, 2018 p. 172.

**But in Western European democracies too, the distribution of economic prosperity in recent decades has been far from even [. . .]**

For figures on the Netherlands, see L. van Noije and J. Iedema, *Achtervolgd door angst* [Haunted by Fear], report by The Nether-lands Institute for Social Research, 2017, p. 81.

**Looking at the specifics: if you are unemployed [. . .] as part of an anxiety disorder.**

R. de Graaf et al., *De psychische gezondheid van de Nederlandse bevolking. NEMESIS-2: Opzet en eerste resultaten* [The Mental Health of the Dutch Population. NEMESIS-2: Design and Initial Results], Trimbos Institute, 2010, p. 104.

**The story of the self-esteem movement (including quotes)**

W. Storr, "'It was quasi-religious': the great self-esteem con", *The Guardian*, 3 June 2017.

W. Storr, *Selfie: How the West Became Self-Obsessed*, 2017.

**In fact, high self-esteem is often [. . .] associated with a lack of empathy and a notorious inability to realistically assess your own abilities.**

L. Slater, "The Trouble with Self-Esteem", *The New York Times Magazine*, 3 February 2002.

J. Kruger and D. Dunning, "Unskilled and Unaware of It: How Difficulties in Recognizing One's Own Incompetence Lead to Inflated Self-assessments", *Journal of Personality and Social Psychology* 77(6), 1999, pp. 1121–1134.

**Yet this culture took root at a time when, in concrete terms, millennials were in considerably worse shape [. . .] on the housing market.**

J.M. Twenge, *Generation Me*, 2014, p. 161.

**Psychologists and sociologists refer to this increase as the "narcissism epidemic".**

E. de Bellis et al., "The Influence of Trait and State Narcissism on the Uniqueness of Mass-Customized Products", *Journal of Retailing* 92(2), 2016, pp. 162–172.

J.M. Twenge and W.K. Campbell, *The Narcissism Epidemic*, 2009.

J.M. Twenge, *Generation Me*, 2014, pp. 30–48.

**This sense of psychological entitlement. . .**

L. Ashner and M. Meyerson, *When Is Enough, Enough? What You Can Do If You Never Feel Satisfied*, 1997, pp. 106–107.

But thanks to the unstoppable force of individualisation, our notions of morality have become detached from what were once their collective sources: religious texts, shared beliefs...

C. Taylor, *Sources of the Self. The Making of the Modern Identity*, 1989.

## On Christian Smith's research

C. Smith, *Lost in Translation. The Dark Side of Emerging Adulthood*, 2011.

Quotes from D. Brooks article "If It Feels Right", *The New York Times*, 12 September 2011.

[...] the percentage of Dutch people who thought norms and values had deteriorated rose from forty to sixty per cent between 1968 and 2006, [...] the highest percentage in almost 30 years.

P. Schnabel, R. Bijl and J. de Hart, *Betrekkelijke betrokkenheid: Studies in sociale cohesie* [Relative Involvement: Studies in Social Cohesion], report by The Netherlands Institute for Social Research, 2008.

## Jan Swinkels on our culture of success

From my conversation with Swinkels in October 2018.

The short circuit created by this colossal mismatch [...] an unprecedented rise in psychiatric disorders throughout the Western world.

P. Verhaeghe, *Identiteit* [Identity], 2012, p. 78.

## Bauman on freedom and powerlessness

P. Verhaeghe, *Identiteit* [Identity], 2012, p. 175.

"Anxiety is essentially feeling a lack of control [...] This mental shift has become very hard for us to achieve [...]"

From an interview on Dutch broadcaster Human's radio show *Brainwash Zomerradio*, 2018.

And a follow-up conversation I had with Denys on 7 July 2019.

All over the world, supposedly impartial bodies [. . .] are coming under intense pressure.

M. Lewis, *Against the Rules*, podcast from 2019.

Western societies are dealing with what French philosopher François Ewald has described as a crisis of causality [. . .]

F. Ewald, "The Return of Descartes's Malicious Demon: An Outline of a Philosophy of Precaution", in T. Baker and J. Simon (eds), *Embracing Risk: The Changing Culture of Insurance and Responsibility*, 2002, pp. 273–301.

F. Ewald, "Insurance and Risk" in G. Burchell, C. Gordon and P. Miller (eds), *The Foucault Effect. Studies in Governmentality*, 1991.

F. Furedi, *Culture of Fear*, 2006, p. 37.

Universal Truth as a universal antidote.

N. van Verschuer, "Hoe angst de wereld veroverde" [How Fear Conquered the World], *NRC Handelsblad*, 27 September 2018.

We live in an impenetrable and complex world, without much in the way of factual guidance. For anxiety, there is no better breeding ground imaginable.

J. Averill, "Disorders of Emotion", *Journal of Social and Clinical Psychology* 6(3–4), 1988, pp. 247–268.

G. Glas, *Concepten van angst en angststoornissen. Een psychiatrische en vakfilosofische study*. [Concepts of Anxiety and Anxiety Disorders: A Psychiatric and Professional Philosophical Study], 1991.

Crime rates in the US and the UK have been falling for years, yet there is a widespread perception that crime is on the rise.

F. Furedi, *Culture of Fear*, 2006.

J.M. Twenge, "The Age of Anxiety? Birth Cohort Change in Anxiety and Neuroticism, 1952–1993", *Journal of Personality and Social Psychology* 79(6), 2000, pp. 1007–1021.

Even in the Netherlands [. . .] 54 per cent of the population believe crime is increasing, though this is by no means the case.

*De sociale staat van Nederland* [The Social State of the Netherlands], report by The Netherlands Institute for Social Research, 2018.

The media reinforce these tendencies [. . .] feelings of helplessness or even despair.

P. Giesen, *Land van lafaards?* [Country of Cowards?], 2007, p. 302.
J.M. Twenge, *Generation Me*, 2014, p. 192.

There is a strong correlation between media consumption and feeling unsafe: the more news you watch and read, the more unsafe you tend to feel.

*Achtervolgd door angst* [Haunted by Fear], report by The Netherlands Institute for Social Research, 2017, p. 86.

Beck even goes one step further, arguing that the primary source of danger is no longer ignorance, as we have assumed for centuries, but knowledge.

U. Beck, *Risk Society: Towards A New Modernity*, 1992, p. 183.

Yet in the early days of online communication [. . .] would become less of an issue.

J.A. Gold, "Does CMC Present Individuals with Disabilities Opportunities or Barriers?" Consulted at www.december.com/cmc/mag/1997/jan/gold.html and cited in P. Schnabel, R. Bijl and J. de Hart, *Betrekkelijke betrokkenheid: Studies in sociale cohesie* [Relative Involvement: Studies in Social Cohesion], report by The Netherlands Institute for Social Research, 2008.

J.E. Katz and P. Aspden, "A nation of strangers?", *Communication of the Association for Computing Machinery* 40(12), 1997, pp. 81–86.

B. Wellman, "From Little Boxes to Loosely Bounded Networks: The Privatization and Domestication of Community" in J.L. Abu-Lughod (ed.), *Sociology for the Twenty-first Century. Continuities and Cutting-Edges*, 1999, pp. 94–114.

**Scientists speak of the Matthew effect [. . .]**

R. van den Eijnden and A. Vermulst, "Online communicatie, compulsief internetgebruik en het psychosociale welbevinden van jongeren" [Online Communication, Compulsive Internet Use and the Psychosocial Well-being of Young People], in J. de Haan and C. van 't Hof (eds), *Jaarboek ICT en samenleving. De digitale generatie* [ICT and Society Yearbook. The Digital Generation], 2006, pp. 25–44.

J. Peter and P.M. Valkenburg, "Research Note. Individual Differences in Perceptions of Internet Communication", *European Journal of Communication* 21(2), 2006, pp. 213–226.

**Dopamine in particular is a pleasurable and addictive hormone, one which – contrary to popular belief – relates primarily to the expectation of reward rather than pleasure itself.**

M. Keulemans, "Een bericht vol dopamine" [A message full of dopamine], *de Volkskrant*, 13 September 2019.

**"Every like is a moment of self-affirmation."**

This quote comes from a Dutch TV interview with Marleen Stekker for the programme *Zomergasten*, 12 August 2018.

**Social media can breed envy and plant seeds of inferiority, seeds that may or may not grow into anxiety or depression.**

J.M. Twenge, *iGen. Why Today's Super-Connected Kids Are Growing Up Less Rebellious, More Tolerant, Less Happy - And Completely Unprepared for Adulthood - And What That Means for the Rest of Us*, 2017, p. 101.

In 2015, over 70 per cent of Western teens had access to a smartphone, an estimate that has surely gone up since.

J.M. Twenge, "Are smartphones causing more teen suicides?", *The Guardian*, 24 May 2018.

The number of American high school students aged fourteen to sixteen who struggle with loneliness increased by 31 per cent between 2012 and 2015.

J.M. Twenge, *iGen*, 2017, p. 97.

The time in which you grow up accounts for an estimated twenty per cent of the difference in anxiety levels across generations.

J. Twenge, *Generation Me*, 2014, p. 145.

## INTERMEZZO: O FEAR, I KNOW THEE

### Quote from John Keats
J. Keats, "Ode on Melancholy" in *The Complete Poems of John Keats*, 2015.

### Quote from William Collins
W. Collins, "Ode to Fear" in R. Lonsdale (ed.), *The Poems of Thomas Gray, William Collins and Oliver Goldsmith*, 1969, pp. 418–423.

## 13 THE CURIOUS CASE OF MICHAEL BERNARD LOGGINS

**Quote from Socrates**

Plato, *Phaedrus*. Translated by W. Hamilton, 1974, pp. 46–47.

**Quote from Aristotle**

Aristotle, *Problems II: Books XXII-XXXVIII*. Translated by W.S. Hett, 1936, pp. 155–157.

**On Aristotle's *Problems***

P. van der Eijk's introduction to his translation *Aristoteles. Over melancholie* [Aristotle: On Melancholy], 2001.

**Quote from Byron**

E.J. Lovell (ed.), *Lady Blessington's Conversations of Lord Byron*, 1969, p. 115. Quoted in: K.R. Jamison, *Touched with Fire*, 1993, p. 2.

**Artists of all countries, eras and disciplines have talked about their inner pain as integral to their work.**

Relevant quotes can be found in E.G. Wilson, *Against Happiness*, 2008, pp. 125, 139, 141, 144.

The quote from Van Gogh: *The Complete Letters of Vincent van Gogh* Vol. II (Letter 514), 1958, p. 620.

The quote from Poe: "Romance" in *The Fall of the House of Usher and Other Writings*, 2003, p. 521.

**Edvard Munch on his "fear of life"**

E. Munch and J.G. Holland (ed.), *We Are Flames Which Pour Out of the Earth. The Private Journals of Edvard Munch*, 2005.

**T.S. Eliot on inspiration**

T.S. Eliot, *The Use of Poetry and the Use of Criticism* (1933), quoted by M. Ford, "I Gotta Use Words", *The London Review of Books* 38(16), 11 August 2016.

## The selection of "crazy" poets is drawn from

K.R. Jamison, *Touched with Fire: Manic-Depressive Illness and the Artistic Temperament*, 1993, pp. 63–71.

## The cited studies on creativity

N.C. Andreasen and A. Canter, "The creative writer: psychiatric symptoms and family history", *Comprehensive Psychiatry* 15, 1974, pp. 123–131.

N.C. Andreasen and P.S. Powers, "Creativity and Psychosis: An Examination of Conceptual Style", *Archives of General Psychiatry* 32, 1975, pp. 70–73.

N.C. Andreasen, "Creativity and Mental Illness: Prevalence Rates in Writers and Their First-degree Relatives", *American Journal of Psychiatry* 144(10), 1987, pp. 1288–1292.

K.R. Jamison, *Touched with Fire*, 1993.

S. Kyaga et al., "Mental Illness, Suicide and Creativity: 40-Year Prospective Total Population Study", *Journal of Psychiatric Research* 47(1), 2013, pp. 83–90.

A.M. Ludwig, "Creative Achievement and Psychopathology: Comparison among Professions", *American Journal of Pychotherapy* 46(3), 1992, pp. 330–354.

C. Martindale, "Father's Absence, Psychopathology, and Poetic Eminence", *Psychological Reports* 31(3), 1972, pp. 843–847.

C. Martindale, *The Clockwork Muse: The Predictability of Artistic Change*, 1990.

R.A. Power et al., "Polygenic Risk Scores for Schizophrenia and Bipolar Disorder Predict Creativity", *Nature Neuroscience* 18(7), 2015, pp. 953–955.

## Hypomania is a condition of intense excitement that sometimes precedes mania.

Based on K.R. Jamison, *Touched with Fire*, 1993.

N.C. Andreasen, *The Creating Brain. The Neuroscience of Genius*, 2005, pp. 31–37, 77–78, 102.

What about the periods of depression, of melancholy and anxiety? What purpose do they serve?

K.R. Jamison, *Touched with Fire*, 1993.

H.A. Sackheim, "Self-deception, Self-esteem and Depression: The Adaptive Value of Lying to Oneself" in J. Masling (ed.), *Empirical Studies of Psychonalytic Theories Vol. 1*, 1983, pp. 101–157.

S.E. Taylor and J.D. Brown, "Illusion and Wellbeing: a Social Psychological Perspective on Mental Health", *Psychological Bulletin* 103, 1988, pp. 193–210.

What exactly is an artist? Writer Tim Parks sees them as people who have never found a stable position between the poles of fear and courage [. . .]

T. Parks, "Fear and Literature", *The New York Review of Books Daily*, 11 May 2012.

## 14 AN ANATOMY OF FAILED CONVERSATIONS

### Quote from Witte Hoogendijk

From a 2009 interview for *Kijken in de ziel*, a series of in-depth TV interviews with leading Dutch psychiatrists and pyschologists.

So it's not so surprising to learn that someone [. . .] with a clean bill of mental health [. . .]

A.J. van Balkom et al., "Comorbidity of the anxiety disorders in a community-based older population in The Netherlands", *Acta Psychiatrica Scandinavica* 101, 2000, pp. 37–45.

A.J. van Balkom et al., "Comorbid depression, but not comorbid anxiety disorders, predicts poor outcome in anxiety disorders", *Depression and Anxiety* 25, 2008, pp. 408–415.

R.M.A. Hirschfeld, "The Comorbidity of Major Depression and Anxiety Disorders: Recognition and Management in Primary

Care", *Primary Care Companion to the Journal of Clinical Psychiatry* 3(6), 2001, pp. 244–254.

J. Sareen et al., "The Relationship between Anxiety Disorders and Physical Disorders in the U.S. National Comorbidity Survey", *Depression and Anxiety* 21(4), 2005, pp. 193–202.

J. Sareen et al., "Anxiety Disorders and Risk for Suicidal Ideation and Suicide Attempts: A Population-based Longitudinal Study of Adults", *Archives of General Psychiatry* 62, 2005, pp. 1249–1257.

## The cover band comparison made by Johann Hari

J. Hari, *Lost Connections*, 2018, p. 15.

## The poem "Sappho 31"

This translation is the work of Chris Childers.

## On Simon Vestdijk

S. Vestdijk, *Het wezen van de angst* [The Essence of Fear], 1968.
An exchange of letters with Vestdijk's biographer Wim Hazeu in February 2019.

## I felt raw, naked, fragile, weary, wasted.

This translation is based on a line from the 2019 Dutch stage adaptation of Georges Perec's novel *Un homme qui dort* by theatre company BOG.

## Quote from Georges Perec

G. Perec, *Things: A Story of the Sixties & A Man Asleep*, 1990, p. 142. Translated by David Bellos and Andrew Leak.

**Professor Denis Noble and Wittgenstein's ladder**
A. Barret, "Face to Face with Denis Noble", *The Oxford Scientist*,
2022.

**Many thanks to my fellow insiders for sharing their metaphors
with me.**
Their full names are on record and all of them have kindly
given me their permission to incorporate their words into this
chapter.

**All passages from Plath's work come from**
S. Plath and K.V. Kukil (ed.), *The Unabridged Journals of Sylvia
Plath*, 2000.
They have been analysed by Z. Demjén in *Sylvia Plath and the
Language of Affective States. Written Discourse and the Experience
of Depression*, 2015.

**Findings such as these have led scholars to view density of meta-
phor as a linguistic indicator of emotional intensity.**
A. Ortony and F. Fainsilber, "The Role of Metaphors in
Descriptions of Emotions", *Proceedings of the 1987 Workshop
on Theoretical Issues in Language Processing*, 1987.

**Psychologist and data scientist Johannes Eichstaedt of the Univer-
sity of Pennsylvania calls this "I Language".**
J.C. Eichstaedt et al., "Facebook language predicts depression in
medical records", *Proceedings of the National Academy of Sciences
of the United States of America*, 115(44), 2018, pp. 11203–11208.

**About Viktor von Gebsattel and alternative realities**
G. Glas, *Angst: Beleving, structuur, macht* [Fear: Perception,
Structure, Power], 2008, pp. 50–51.
D. Leader, *What is Madness?*, 2012.

**Hanson was telling a friend about a conversation he'd had while out walking one day.**

The conversation in the park between Todd Hanson and his friend is from Marc Maron's book *Waiting for the Punch*, 2018.

**Which is why there are such strong similarities in the feelings colours evoke across various cultures.**

F. Adams and C. Osgood, "A Cross-Cultural Study of the Affective Meaning of Color", *Journal of Cross-Cultural Psychology* 4, 1973, pp. 135–156.

**Around the world, in all age groups, white prompts positive associations and black tends towards negative.**

E.B. Shiraev and D. Levy, *Cross-cultural Psychology. Critical Thinking and Contemporary Applications*, 2001.

**I have not been able to trace the exact source of this quote by Stephen Fry. But if their online profile is anything to go by, there can be little doubt that these noble sentiments, eloquently expressed, are his.**

## 16 MOTHER OF DRAGONS

**In reality, the exceptions – those who officially suffer from a disorder – are at a point a little further from the mean, nothing more.**

R. Plomin, *Blueprint*, 2018, pp. 55–65.

W. Hoogendijk and W. de Rek, *Van big bang tot burn-out. Het grote verhaal over stress* [From Big Bang to Burnout: The Big Story about Stress], 2017, p. 230.

**A condition such as haemochromatosis [. . .] would not have survived the Ice Age.**

S. Kurbel, "Was the Last Ice Age dusty climate instrumental in spreading of the three 'Celtic' diseases (hemochromatosis, cystic fibrosis and palmar fibromatosis)?", *Medical Hypotheses* 122, 2019, pp. 134–138.

K.M. Heath et al., "The evolutionary adaptation of the C282Y mutation to culture and climate during the European Neolithic", *American Journal of Physical Anthropology* 160(1), 2016, pp. 86–101.

S. Blakeslee, "New Theory Places Origin of Diabetes in an Age of Icy Hardships", *The New York Times*, 17 May 2005.

**According to the DSM and the doctors who rely on it [. . .] a life without side effects.**

R. Aviv, "The Challenge of Going Off Psychiatric Drugs", *The New Yorker*, 1 April 2019.

**[. . .] qualities you can hone by proving to yourself and others that you can handle situations despite feelings of anxiety, not by seeking to dispel them at all costs.**

A. Bandura, "Self-efficacy: toward a unifying theory of behavioral change", *Psychological Review* 84, 1978, pp. 191–215.

**Recent research at the University of Groningen [. . .] Autonomy pays.**

A. Hovenkamp-Hermelink, "The long-term course of anxiety disorders: An epidemiological perspective", PhD thesis defended at the University of Groningen on 21 December 2020.

**In 1997, Professor Sheila Mehta of Auburn University in the US state of Alabama conducted an interesting study [. . .] less kindly towards them.**

Quoted in J. Hari, *Lost Connections*, 2018, pp. 187–188.

**Could a diagnosis be characterised as "a cluster of behavioural traits"?**

I.D. Yalom, *Love's Executioner and Other Tales of Psychotherapy*, 1989, p. 185.

**The quote from Jeanette Winterson comes from**
*Why Be Happy When You Could Be Normal*, 2011, p. 221.

**Natalie Diaz's poem**
"From the Desire Field" was originally published in Poem-a-Day on 5 June 2017 by the Academy of American Poets (poets.org).

DAAN HEERMA VAN VOSS has written for a number of national and international newspapers, including *The New York Times*, *Vogue US*, *Pen International*, *Haaretz* and *Svenska Dagbladet*. His novels have been shortlisted for several literary prizes and he was awarded De Tegel for extraordinary journalistic achievement. *The Anxiety Project* is his first major work of nonfiction.

DAVID DOHERTY studied English and literary linguistics in Glasgow before moving to Amsterdam, where he has been working as a translator for over twenty years. His translation of Jaap Robben's *Zomervacht* won the 2021 Vondel Translation Prize and was longlisted for the 2021 International Booker Prize.